P
THE

Gerald Durrell was b   in 1925.
In 1928 his family returned to England and in 1933
they went to live on the Continent. Eventually they
settled on the island of Corfu, where they lived until
1939. During this time he made a special study of
zoology, and kept a large number of the local wild
animals as pets. In 1945 he joined the staff of Whipsnade
Park as a student keeper. In 1947 he financed,
organized, and led his first animal-collecting expedition to the Cameroons. This was followed by a
second expedition in 1948 and a third in 1949, this
time to British Guiana. He has also made expeditions
to Paraguay, Argentina and Sierra Leone. In 1962 he
and his wife went to New Zealand, Australia, and
Malaya to film a TV series, *Two in the Bush*, in con-
junction with the BBC Natural History Film Unit.
       he founded the Jersey Zoological Park, of
which he is the director, and in 1964 he founded the
Jersey Wildlife Preservation Trust. Gerald Durrell's
other books include *My Family and Other Animals,
Encounters with Animals, Three Singles to Adventure,
A Zoo in My Luggage, The Whispering Land, The
Drunken Forest, Menagerie Manor, Birds, Beasts and
Relatives, Fillets of Plaice, Catch Me a Colobus, Beasts
in My Belfry, The Talking Parcel, The Stationary Ark,
Golden Bats and Pink Pigeons, Garden of the Gods, Picnic
and Suchlike Pandemonium*, and, with Lee Durrell, *The
Amateur Naturalist*.

GERALD DURRELL

THE BAFUT BEAGLES

WITH ILLUSTRATIONS BY
Ralph Thompson

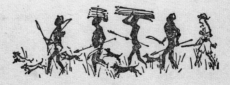

PENGUIN BOOKS

Penguin Books Ltd, 27 Wrights Lane, London w8 5tz (Publishing and Editorial)
and Harmondsworth, Middlesex, England (Distribution and Warehouse)
Viking Penguin Inc., 40 West 23rd Street, New York, New York 10010, USA
Penguin Books Australia Ltd, Ringwood, Victoria, Australia
Penguin Books Canada Ltd, 2801 John Street, Markham, Ontario, Canada L3R 1B4
Penguin Books (N.Z.) Ltd, 182–190 Wairau Road, Auckland 10, New Zealand

First published by Rupert Hart Davis 1954
Published in Penguin Books 1958
Reprinted 1959, 1961 (twice), 1963, 1964, 1965, 1967, 1968, 1970, 1971 (twice),
1972, 1973, 1974, 1975, 1977, 1978, 1979, 1981, 1982, 1984, 1986, 1988

Made and printed in Great Britain
by Richard Clay Bungay, Suffolk
Set in Monotype Garamond

CONTENTS

In Which We Done Come

THE Cross River picks its way down from the mountains of the Cameroons, until it runs sprawling and glittering into the great bowl of forest land around Mamfe. After being all froth, waterfalls, and eager chattering in the mountains, it settles down when it reaches this forest, and runs sedately in its rocky bed, the gently moving waters creating ribs of pure white sand across its width, and washing the mud away from the tree roots, so that they look as though they stand at the edge of the water on a tangled, writhing mass of octopus-like legs. It moves along majestically, its brown waters full of hippo and crocodile, and the warm air above it filled with hawking swallows, blue and orange and white.

Just above Mamfe the river increases its pace slightly, squeezing itself between two high rocky cliffs, cliffs that are worn smooth by the passing waters and wear a tattered antimacassar of undergrowth that hangs down from the forest above; emerging from the gorge it swirls out into a vast egg-shaped basin. A little further along, through an identical gorge, another river empties itself into this same basin, and the waters meet and mix in a skein of tiny currents, whirlpools, and ripples, and then continue onwards as one waterway, leaving, as a result of their marriage, a huge glittering hummock of white sand in the centre of the river, sand that is pockmarked with the footprints of hippo and patterned with chains of bird-tracks. Near this island of sand the forest on the bank gives way to the small grassfield that surrounds the village of

Mamfe, and it was here, on the edge of the forest, above the smooth brown river, that we chose to have our base camp.

It took two days of cutting and levelling to get the camp site ready, and on the third day Smith and I stood at the edge of the grassfield watching while thirty sweating, shouting Africans hauled and pulled at what appeared to be the vast, brown, wrinkled carcass of a whale that lay on the freshly turned red earth. Gradually, as this sea of canvas was pulled and pushed, it rose into the air, swelling like an unhealthy looking puffball. Then it seemed to spread out suddenly, leechlike, and turned itself into a marquee of impressive dimensions. When it had thus revealed its identity, there came a full-throated roar, a mixture of astonishment, amazement, and delight, from the crowd of villagers who had come to watch our camp building.

Once the marquee was ready to house us, it took another week of hard work before we were ready to start collecting. Cages had to be erected, ponds dug, various chiefs from nearby villages interviewed and told of the animals we required, food supplies had to be laid on, and a hundred and one other things had to be done. Eventually, when the camp was functioning smoothly, we felt we could start collecting in earnest. We had decided that Smith should stay in Mamfe and keep the base camp going, gleaning what forest fauna he could with the help of the local inhabitants, while I was to travel further inland to the mountains, where the forest gave place to the great grasslands. In this mountain world, with its strange vegetation and cooler climate, a completely different fauna from that of the steamy forest region was to be found.

I was not certain which part of the grasslands would be the best for me to operate in, so I went to the District Officer for advice. I explained my dilemma, and he produced a map of the mountains and together we pored over it. Suddenly he dabbed his forefinger down and glanced at me.

'What about Bafut?' he asked.

'Is that a good place? What are the people like?'

'There is only one person you have to worry about in Bafut, and that's the Fon,' he said; 'get him on your side and the people will help you all they can.'

'Is he the chief?'

'He's the sort of Nero of this region,' said the D.O., marking a large circle on the map with his finger, 'and what he says goes. He's the most delightful old rogue, and the quickest and surest way to his heart is to prove to him that you can carry your liquor. He's got a wonderful great villa there, which he built in case he had any European visitors, and I'm sure if you wrote to him he would let you stay there. It's worth a visit, is Bafut, even if you don't stay.'

'Well, I'll drop him a note and see what he says.'

'See that your communication is . . . er . . . well lubricated,' said the D.O.

'I'll go down to the store and get a bottle of lubrication at once,' I assured him.

So that afternoon, a messenger went off to the mountains, carrying with him my note and a bottle of gin. Four days later he returned, bearing a letter from the Fon, a masterly document that encouraged me tremendously.

> Fon's Office Bafut, Bafut Bemenda Division,
> 5th March, 1949.

My good friend,

Yours of 3rd March, 1949, came in hand with all contents well marked out.

Yes, I accept your arrival to Bafut in course of two month stay about your animals and too, I shall be overjoyed to let you be in possession of a house in my compound if you will do well in arrangement of rentages.

> Yours cordially,
> Fon of Bafut.

I made arrangements to leave for Bafut at once.

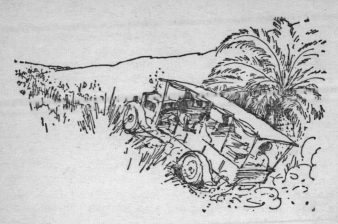

CHAPTER ONE

Toads and Dancing Monkeys

MOST West African lorries are not in what one would call the first flush of youth, and I had learnt by bitter experience not to expect anything very much of them. But the lorry that arrived to take me up to the mountains was worse than anything I had seen before: it tottered on the borders of senile decay. It stood there on buckled wheels, wheezing and gasping with exhaustion from having to climb up the gentle slope to the camp, and I consigned myself and my loads to it with some trepidation. The driver, who was a cheerful fellow, pointed out that he would require my assistance in two very necessary operations: first, I had to keep the hand brake pressed down when travelling downhill, for unless it was held thus almost level with the floor it sullenly refused to function. Secondly, I had to keep a stern eye on the clutch, a wilful piece of mechanism, that seized every chance to leap out of its socket with a noise like a strangling leopard. As it was obvious that not even a West African lorry driver could be successful in driving while crouched under the dashboard in a pre-natal position, I had to take over control of these instruments if I valued my life. So, while I ducked at intervals to put on the brake, amid the rich smell of

12

burning rubber, our noble lorry jerked its way towards the mountains at a steady twenty miles per hour; sometimes, when a downward slope favoured it, it threw caution to the winds and careered along in a madcap fashion at twenty-five.

For the first thirty miles the red earth road wound its way through the lowland forest, the giant trees standing in solid ranks alongside and their branches entwined in an archway of leaves above us. Flocks of hornbills flapped across the road, honking like the ghosts of ancient taxis, and on the banks, draped decoratively in the patches of sunlight, the agama lizards lay, blushing into sunset colouring with excitement and nodding their heads furiously. Slowly and almost imperceptibly the road started to climb upwards, looping its way in languid curves round the forested hills. In the back of the lorry the boys lifted up their voices in song:

> *Home again, home again,*
> *When shall I see ma home?*
> *When shall I see ma mammy?*
> *I'll never forget ma home . . .*

The driver hummed the refrain softly to himself, glancing at me to see if I would object. To his surprise I joined in, and so while the lorry rolled onwards trailing a swirling tail of red dust behind it, the boys in the back maintained the chorus while the driver and I harmonized and sang complicated twiddly bits, and the driver played a staccato accompaniment on the horn.

Breaks in the forest became more frequent the higher we climbed, and presently a new type of undergrowth began to appear: massive tree-ferns standing in conspiratorial groups at the roadside on their thick, squat, and hairy trunks, the fronds of leaves sprouting from the tops like delicate green fountains. These ferns were the guardians of a new world, for suddenly, as though the hills had shrugged themselves free of a cloak, the forest disappeared. It lay behind us in the valley, a thick pelt of green undulating away into the heat-shimmered distance, while above us the hillside rose majestically, covered in a coat of rippling, waist-high grass, bleached golden by the sun. The lorry crept higher and higher, the engine gasping and shuddering with this unaccustomed activity. I began to think that we should have to push the wretched thing up the last two or three hundred feet, but to everyone's surprise we made it, and the lorry crept on to the brow of the hill, trembling with fatigue, spouting steam from its radiator like a dying whale. We crawled to a standstill and the driver switched off the engine.

'We go wait small-time, engine get hot,' he explained, pointing to the forequarters of the lorry, which were by now completely invisible under a cloud of steam. Thankfully I descended from the red-hot inside of the cab and strolled down to where the road dipped into the next valley. From this vantage point I could see the country we had travelled through and the country we were about to enter.

Behind lay the vast green forest, looking from this distance as tight and impenetrable as lambs' wool; only on the hilltops was there any apparent break in the smooth surface of those millions of leaves, for against the sky the trees were silhouetted in a tattered fringe. Ahead of us lay a world so different that it seemed incredible that the two should be found side by side. There was no gradual merging: behind lay the forest of huge trees, each clad in its robe of polished leaves, glittering like green and gigantic pearly kings; ahead, to the furthermost dim blue horizon, lay range after range of hills, merging and folding into one another like great frozen waves, tilting their faces to the sun, covered from valley to crest with a rippling fur of golden-green grass that paled or darkened as the wind curved and smoothed it. Behind us the forest was decked out in the most vivid of greens and scarlets – harsh and intense colours. Before us, in this strange mountain world of grass, the colours were soft and delicate – fawns, pale greens, warm browns, and golds. The smoothly crumpled hills covered with this pastel-tinted grass could have been an English scene: the downland country of the south on a larger scale. The illusion was spoilt, however, by the sun, which shone fiercely and steadily in a completely un-English manner.

From then onwards the road resembled a switchback, and we rattled and squeaked our way down into valleys, and coughed and grunted our way up the steep hillsides. We had paused on one hilltop to let the engine cool again, and I noticed in the valley ahead a village, looking at that distance like an irregular patch of black toadstools against the green. When the engine was switched off, the silence descended like a blanket; all we could hear was the soft hiss of the grass moved by the wind and, from the village far below us, the barking of a dog and the crowing of a cockerel, the sounds tiny and remote but clear as a bell. Through my field-glasses I could see that there was some activity going on in the village: crowds of people milled round the huts, and I could see the flash of machetes and spears, and the occasional glint of a gaudy sarong.

'Na whatee dat palaver for dat place?' I asked the driver.

He peered down the hill, screwing up his eyes, and then turned to me, grinning delightedly.

'Na market, sah,' he explained, and then, hopefully. 'Masa want to stop for dat place?'

'You tink sometime we go find beef for sale dere?'

'Yes, sah!'

'For true?'

'For true, sah!'

'You lie, bushman,' I said in mock anger. 'You want to stop for dis place so you go find corn beer. No be so?'

'Eh! Na so, sah,' admitted the driver, smiling, 'but sometimes Masa go find beef there also.'

'All right, we go stop small time.'

'Yes, sah,' said the driver eagerly, and sent the lorry hurtling down the slope towards the village.

The big huts, with their conical thatched roofs, were grouped neatly round a small square which was shaded with groups of young eucalyptus trees. In this square was the market; in the patchwork of light and shadow under the slim trees the traders had spread their wares on the ground, each on his own little patch, and around them thronged the villagers in a gesticulating, chattering, arguing wedge. The wares offered for sale were astonishing in their variety and, sometimes, in their incongruity. There were freshwater catfish, dried by wood smoke and spitted on short sticks. These are unpleasant-looking fish when alive, but when dried and shrivelled and blackened by the smoking they looked like some fiendish little juju dolls, twisted into strange contortions by a revolting dance. There were great bales of cloth, some of it the highly coloured prints so beloved of the African, imported from England; more tasteful was the locally woven cloth, thick and soft. Among these patches of highly coloured cloth were an odd assortment of eggs, chickens in bamboo baskets, green peppers, cabbages, potatoes, sugar-cane, great gory hunks of meat, giant Cane Rats, neatly gutted and hung on strings, earthenware pots and cane baskets, eroco-wood chairs, needles, gunpowder, corn beer, gin-traps, mangoes, pawpaws, enemas, lemons, native shoes, lovely raffia-work bags, nails, flints, carbide and cascara, spades and leopard skins, plimsolls, trilbys, calabashes full of palm wine, and old kerosene tins full of palm and groundnut oil.

The inhabitants of the market were as varied and as curious as the wares offered for sale: there were Hausa men clad in their brilliant white robes and little white skull-caps; local chieftains in multi-coloured robes and richly embroidered caps with tassels; there were the pagans from distant mountain villages, wearing nothing but a scrap of dirty leather round the loins, their teeth filed to points, their faces tattooed. For them this represented a teeming metropolis, and the market was perhaps the high spot of the year's amusements. They argued fiercely, waving their arms, pushing each other, their dark eyes shining with delight, over such things as cocoa yams or Cane Rats; or else they stood in little groups gazing with hopeless longing at the toppling piles of multi-coloured cloth, milling round from one vantage point to another, in order to get the best views of these unobtainable luxuries.

My staff and the lorry driver disappeared into this pungent, swirling crowd like ants into a treacle tin, and I was left to wander round by myself. After a time I decided to try to take some photographs of the pagan tribesmen, so I set up the camera and started to focus it. Immediately, pandemonium broke loose; the tribesmen with one accord dropped their goods and chattels and fled for the nearest shelter, screaming wildly. Rather bewildered by this, for the average African is generally only too pleased to have his photograph taken, I turned to a Hausa standing close by and asked him what was the matter. The explanation was interesting: apparently the pagans knew what a camera was, and knew that it produced pictures of the people it was pointed at. But they were firmly convinced that with each photograph taken the photographer gained a small portion of his subject's soul, and if he took many photographs he would gain complete control over the person in question. This is a good example of witchcraft being brought up to date; in the old days if you obtained some of your victim's hair or toe-nails you had great power over him; nowadays if you get a photograph it apparently acts just as well. However, in spite of the reluctance on the parts of my subjects, I did manage to get a few shots of them, by the simple method of standing sideways on, looking in the opposite direction, and taking the photographs from under my arm.

It was not long before I discovered something that drove all thoughts of photography and witchcraft out of my head. In one of the dark little stalls that lined the square I caught a flash of reddish fur, and, moving over to investigate, I found the most delightful monkey on the end of a long string, squatting in the dust and uttering loud and penetrating 'prroup' noises. She had light ginger-coloured fur, a white shirt-front, and a mournful black face, and the strange noises she was making sounded like a cross between a bird cry and the friendly greetings of a cat. She sat and watched me very intently for a few seconds, and then she got up suddenly and started to dance. First she rose on her hind legs and jumped up and down vigorously, holding her long arms wide apart, as though she were going to clasp me to her bosom. Then she got down on all fours and started to bounce like a ball, all four feet leaving the ground, her jumps getting higher and higher the more excited she became. Then she stopped and had a short rest before starting on the next part of the dance; this consisted of standing on all fours, keeping her hindquarters quite still, while she flung her forequarters from side to side like a pendulum.

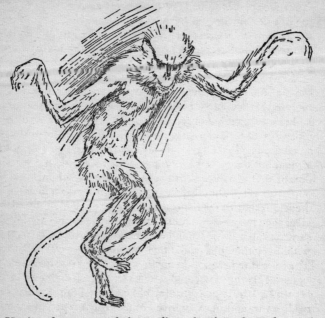

Having demonstrated the outline, she then showed me what could be done by a really experienced dancing monkey, and she twirled and leapt and bounced until I felt quite dizzy. I had been attracted to her from the first, but this wild dervish dance was irresistible, and I felt that I simply had to buy her. I paid her owner twice what she was worth and carried her off triumphantly. I bought her a bunch of bananas at one of the stalls, and she was so overcome by my generosity that she repaid me by wetting all down the front of my shirt. I rounded up the staff and the driver, all breathing corn beer, and we climbed into the lorry and continued our journey. The monkey sat on my knee, stuffing her mouth with bananas and uttering little cries of excitement and pleasure as she watched the scenery out of the window. In view of her accomplishment, I decided to call her Pavlova, and Pavlova the Patas monkey she became forthwith.

We drove on for some hours, and by the time we were nearing our destination the valleys were washed with deep purple shadows and the sun was sinking leisurely into a thousand scarlet-and-green feathers of cloud behind the highest range of western hills.

We knew when we reached Bafut, for there the road ended. On our left lay an enormous dusty courtyard surrounded by a high red brick wall. Behind this was a great assembly of circular huts with high thatched roofs, clustered round a small, neat villa. But all these structures were dominated and dwarfed by an edifice that looked like an old-fashioned bee-hive, magnified a thousand times. It was a huge circular hut, with a massive domed roof of thatch, black and mysterious with age. On the opposite side of the road the ground rose steeply, and a wide flight of some seventy steps curved upwards to another large villa, shoe-box shaped, its upper and lower storeys completely surrounded by wide verandas, the pillars of which were hung with bougainvillaea and other creepers in great profusion. This, I realized, was to be my home for the next few months.

As I got stiffly out of the lorry, an arched doorway in the far wall of the large courtyard opened and a small procession made its way across to where I stood. It consisted of a group of men, most of them elderly, clad in flowing multi-coloured robes that swished as they moved; on their heads they wore little skull-caps which were thickly embroidered in a riot of coloured wools. In the midst of this group walked a tall, slim man with a lively and humorous face. He was dressed in a plain white robe, and his skull-cap was innocent of decoration, yet, in spite of this lack of colour, I at once singled him out as the only one of any importance in the little cavalcade, so regal was his manner. He was the Fon of Bafut, ruler of the great grassland kingdom we had been travelling through and its immense population of black subjects. He was enormously wealthy, and he ruled his kingdom, I knew, with an intelligent, if slightly despotic, cunning. He stopped in front of me, smiling gently, and extended a large and slender hand.

'Welcome,' he said.

It was not until later that I learnt he could speak pidgin

English as well as any of his subjects, but for some reason he was shy of his accomplishment, so we talked through an interpreter who stood, bent deferentially, translating my speech of welcome through his cupped hands. The Fon listened politely while my speech was translated, and then he waved one huge hand at the villa on top of the slope above us.

'Foine!' he said, grinning.

We shook hands again, then he walked back across the courtyard with his councillors and disappeared through the arched doorway, leaving me to install myself in his 'foine' house.

Some two hours later, when I had bathed and eaten, a messenger arrived and informed me that the Fon would like to visit me for a chat if I had sufficiently 'calmed' myself after my journey. I sent back a reply to the effect that I was quite calmed and that I would be delighted to receive a visit from the Fon; then I got out the whisky and awaited his coming. Presently he arrived, accompanied by his small retinue, and we sat on the veranda in the lamplight and talked. I drank his health in whisky and water, and he drank mine in neat whisky. We talked, at first, through an interpreter, but as the level of the whisky fell the Fon started to speak pidgin English. For two hours I was fully occupied in explaining my mission in his country: I brought out books and photographs of the animals I wanted, I drew them on bits of paper and made noises like them when all else failed, and all the time the Fon's glass was being replenished with frightening regularity.

He said that he thought I should be able to get most of the animals I had shown him, and he promised that the next day he would send some good hunters to work for me. But, he went on, the best thing for him to do was to spread the word among his people so that they would all try to 'catch beef' for me; the best opportunity for this, he explained, was in about ten days' time. Then there was to be a certain ceremony: apparently his subjects, on an appointed day, gathered large quantities of dry grass from the hills and valleys and brought it into Bafut so that the Fon could re-thatch the roof of the great juju house and the roofs of his innumerable wives' houses. When the grass had been brought in he provided the food and drink for a feast.

There would be many hundreds of people at this ceremony, assembled from all over the surrounding countryside, and the Fon explained that this would be an ideal opportunity for him to make a speech and explain to his people what I wanted. I agreed heartily, thanked him profusely, and refilled his empty glass. The level in the bottle fell lower and lower, until it was obviously innocent of even the most reluctant drops of liquid. The Fon rose majestically to his feet, stifled a hiccup, and then held out a hand.

'I go!' he proclaimed, waving in the vague direction of his small villa.

'I'm sorry too much,' I said politely; 'you like I go walk for road with you?'

'Yes, my friend,' he beamed. 'Na foine!'

I called for a member of the staff, who came running at the double carrying a hurricane lantern. He preceded us as we walked down the veranda towards the steps. The Fon was still clasping my hand in his, while with the other he gestured at the veranda, the rooms, and the moonlit garden some thirty feet below, muttering 'Foine, foine,' to himself in a self-satisfied way. When we reached the top of the long flight of steps he paused and stared at me pensively for a moment, then he pointed downwards with one long arm:

'Sheventy-foif step,' he beamed.

'Very fine,' I agreed, nodding.

'We go count um,' said the Fon, delighted at the idea. 'Sheventy-foif, we go count um.'

He draped a long arm around my shoulders, leant heavily upon me, and we descended to the road below, counting loudly. As he could not remember the English for any number higher than six we got somewhat confused half-way down, and on reaching the bottom we found that according to the Fon's reckoning there were three steps missing.

'Sheventy-two?' he asked himself; 'no, na, sheventy-foif. Which side dey done go?'

He glared fiercely at his cringing retinue, who were waiting in the road, as though he suspected them of having secreted the missing steps under their robes. Hastily I suggested that we should count them again. We climbed up to the veranda once more, counting wildly, and then, to make quite sure, we counted them all the way down again. The Fon kept counting up to six and then starting again, and I could see that unless something was done we should spend all night searching for the missing steps; so, when we reached the top, and again when we got to the bottom, I said 'Seventy-five!' in loud, triumphant tones, and beamed at my companion. He was a bit reluctant to accept my reckoning at first, for he had only got up to five, and he felt that the missing seventy needed some explaining. However, I assured him that I had won innumerable prizes for mental arithmetic in my youth, and that my total was the correct one. He clasped me to his chest, clutched my hand and wrung it, muttering 'Foine, foine, my friend,' and then wended his way across the great courtyard to his own residence, leaving me to crawl up the seventy-five steps to bed.

The next day, in between coping with a headache brought on by my session with the Fon, I was kept busy building cages for the flood of specimens that I hoped would soon be rolling in. At noon four tall and impressive-looking young men turned ed up, clad in their best and brightest sarongs, and carrying flintlocks. These fearsome weapons were incredibly ancient, and their barrels were pitted and eroded with rust holes, as though each gun had suffered an acute attack of smallpox. I got them to stack these dangerous-looking weapons outside the gate before they came in and talked to me. They were the hunters the Fon had sent, and for half an hour I sat and showed them pictures of animals and explained how much I would pay for the various creatures. Then I told them to go away and spend the afternoon hunting, and to return in the evening with anything they caught. If they caught nothing they were to come again early the following morning. Then I distributed cigarettes, and they wandered off down the road, talking earnestly to each other, and pointing their guns in all directions with great abandon.

That evening one of the four young men turned up again carrying a small basket. He squatted down and gazed at me

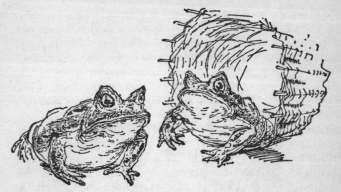

sorrowfully while he explained that he and his companions had not had very good luck with their hunting. They had been a considerable distance, he said, but had found none of the animals I had shown them. However, they had got *something*.

Here he leant forward and put the basket at my feet.

'I no savvay if Masa want dis kind of beef,' he said.

I removed the lid of the basket and peered inside. I thought that it might contain a squirrel, or possibly a rat, but there sat a pair of large and beautiful toads.

'Masa like dis kind of beef?' asked the hunter, watching my face anxiously.

'Yes I like um too much,' I said, and he grinned.

I paid him the required sum of money, 'dashed' him some cigarettes, and he went off, promising to return the following morning with his companions. When he had gone I could turn my attention back to the toads. They were each about the circumference of a saucer, with enormous liquid eyes and short, fat legs that seemed to have some difficulty in supporting their heavy bodies. Their coloration was amazing: their backs were a rich cream, sprinkled with minute black vermiculations; the sides of the heads and bodies were a deep red, a colour that was a cross between mahogany and wine. On their bellies this was replaced by a vivid buttercup yellow.

Now I have always liked toads, for I have found them to be quiet, well-behaved creatures with a charm of their own; they have not the wildly excitable and rather oafish character of the frog, nor his gulping and moist appearance. But, until I met these two, I had always imagined that all toads were pretty much the same, and that having met one you had met them all as far as personality was concerned, though they might differ much in colour and appearance. But I very soon found out that these two amphibians had personalities so striking that they might almost have been mammals.

These creatures are called Brow-leaf Toads, because the curious cream-coloured marking on the back is, in shape and colour, exactly like a dead and withered leaf. If the toad crouches down on the floor of the forest it merges into its background perfectly. Hence its English title; its scientific title is 'Eyebrow Toad', which in Latin sounds even more apt: *Bufo superciliarus*, for the Brow-leaf, on first acquaintance, gives the impression of being overwhelmingly supercilious. Above its large eyes the skin is hitched up into two little points, so that the creature has its eyebrows raised at the world in a markedly sardonic manner. The immensely wide mouth adds to this impression of aristocratic conceit by drooping gently at the corners, thus giving the toad a faintly sneering expression that can only be achieved by one other animal that I know of, the camel. Add to this the slow, swaggering walk, and the fact that the creature squats down every two or three steps and gazes at you with a sort of pitying disdain, and you begin to feel that superciliousness could not go much farther.

My two Brow-leafs squatted side by side on a bed of fresh grass in the bottom of the basket and gazed up at me with expressions of withering scorn. I tipped the basket on its side, and they waddled out on to the floor with all the indignation and dignity of a couple of Lord Mayors who had been accidentally locked in a public lavatory. They walked about three feet across the floor and then, apparently exhausted by this effort, squatted down, gulping gently. They surveyed me very fixedly for some ten minutes with what appeared to be ever-increasing disgust. Then one of them wandered away and eventually crouched down by the leg of the table, evidently under the mistaken impression that it was the trunk of a tree. The other continued to stare at me, and after mature reflection he summed up his opinion of my worth by being sick, bringing up the semi-digested corpses of a grasshopper and two moths. Then he gave me a pained and reproachful look and joined his friend under the table.

As I had no suitable cage ready for them, the Brow-leafs spent the first few days locked in my bedroom, wandering slowly and meditatively about the floor, or squatting in a trance-like state under my bed, and affording me untold amusement by their actions. I discovered, after a few hours' acquaintance with my plump room-mates, that I had sadly misjudged them, for they were not the arrogant, conceited creatures they pretended to be. They were actually shy and easily embarrassed beasts, completely lacking in self-confidence; I suspect that they suffered from deep and ineradicable inferiority complexes and that their insufferable air of superiority was merely a pose to hide from the world the hideous truth, that they had no faith in their fat selves. I discovered this quite by accident the night of their arrival. I was making notes on their coloration, while the toads squatted on the floor at my feet, looking as though they were composing their own entries for Burke's *Peerage*. Wanting to examine their hindquarters more closely, I bent down and picked up one of them between finger and thumb, holding him under the arm-pits, so that he dangled in the air in a most undignified manner. He uttered a loud indignant belch at this treatment and kicked out with his fat hind legs, but my grip was too strong for him and he just had to dangle there until I had finished my examination of his lower regions. Eventually, when I replaced him on the ground next to his companion, he was a different toad altogether. Gone was his aristocratic expression: he was a deflated and humble amphibian. He crouched down, blinking his great eyes nervously, while a sad and timid expression spread over his face. He looked almost as if he was going to cry. This transformation was so sudden and complete that it was astonishing, and I felt absurdly guilty at having been the cause of his ignominy. In order to even things up a bit, I picked up the other one and let him dangle for a while, and he, too, lost his self-confidence and became timid and embarrassed when I replaced him on the floor. They sat there looking so dejected and miserable that it was ludicrous, and my unmannerly laughter proved too much for their sensitive natures, for they waddled rapidly away and hid under the table for the next half-hour. But now that I had learnt their secret I could deflate them at will when they became too haughty: all I had to do was to rap them gently on the nose with my finger, and they would crouch down guiltily, looking as though they were about to blush, and gaze at me with pleading eyes.

I built a nice large cage for my Brow-leafs, and they settled down in it quite happily; however, to keep them healthy, I allowed them to have a walk in the garden every day. When the collection increased, I found that there was too much work to be done for me to be able to stand around patiently while my two blue-blooded aristocrats took the air; I had to cut down on their walks, much to their annoyance. Then, one day, I found a guardian for them in whose hands I could safely leave them while I got on with my work. This guardian was none other than Pavlova the Patas monkey.

Pavlova was extremely tame and gentle, and she took an intense interest in everything that went on around her. The first time I put the Brow-leafs out for a walk near her she was quite captivated by them and stood up on her hind legs, craning her neck to get a better view as they walked sedately across the compound. Going back ten minutes later to see how the toads were getting on, I found that they had both wandered close to the spot where Pavlova was tied. She was squatting between them, stroking them gently with her hands, and uttering loud purring cries of astonishment and pleasure. The toads had the most ridiculously, self-satisfied expressions on their faces, and they were sitting there unmoving, apparently flattered and soothed by her caresses.

Every day after that I would put the toads out near to the place where Pavlova was tied, and she would watch them wandering about. She would give occasional cries of amazement at the sight of them, or else stroke them gently until they lay there in a semi-hypnotized condition. If ever they wandered too far

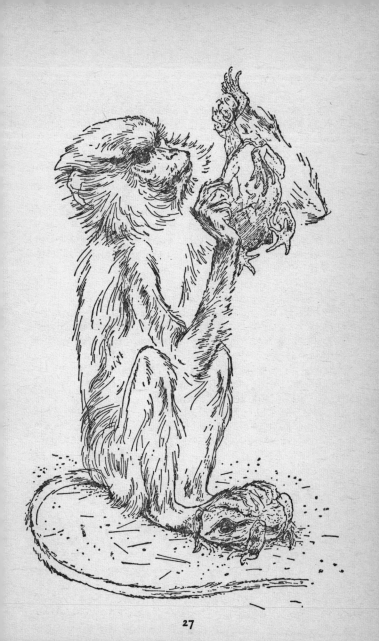

away and were in danger of disappearing into the thick under-growth at the edge of the compound, Pavlova would get very excited and call me with shrill screams to let me know that her charges were escaping, and I would hurry down and bring them back to her. One day she called me when the toads had wandered too far afield, but I did not hear her, and when I went down some time later Pavlova was dancing hysterically at the end of her string, screaming furiously, and the Brow-leafs were nowhere to be seen. I undid the monkey's leash, and she at once led me towards the thick bushes at the edge of the compound, and within a very short time she had found the runaways and had fallen on them with loud purring cries of joy.

Pavlova really got terribly fond of these fat toads, and it was quite touching to see how eagerly she greeted them in the morn-ing, gently stroking and patting them, and how worried she got when they wandered too far away. A thing that she found very difficult to understand was why the toads were not clad in fur, as another monkey would be. She would touch their smooth skins with her fingers, endeavouring to part the non-existent fur, a worried expression on her little black face; oc-casionally she would bend down and lick their backs in a thoughtful sort of way. Eventually she ceased to worry over their baldness, and treated them with the same gentleness and affection she would have displayed towards offspring of her own. The toads, in their own curious way, seemed to become quite fond of her as well, though she sometimes upset their dig-nity, which annoyed them. I remember one morning I had just given them both a bath, which they thoroughly enjoyed, and on walking across the compound they got various bits of stick and dirt stuck to their wet tummies. This worried Pavlova, for she liked her protégés to be clean and neat. I found her sitting in the sunshine, her feet resting on the back of one Brow-leaf as though he were a footstool, while the other one dangled in the most undignified fashion from her hand. As he slowly re-volved in mid-air, Pavlova solemnly picked all the bits of rub-bish from his tummy, talking to him all the time in a series of squeaks and trills. When she had finished with him she put him on the ground, where he sat looking very crestfallen, while his partner was hoisted up into the air and forced to undergo the same indignity. The poor Brow-leafs had no chance of being superior and pompous when Pavlova was around.

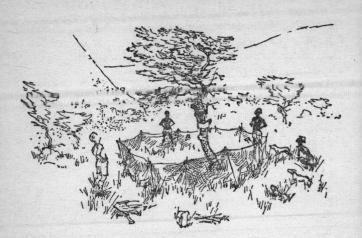

CHAPTER TWO

The Bafut Beagles

IN order to hunt for the various members of the Bafut fauna, I employed, as well as the four hunters the Fon had supplied, a pack of six thin and ungainly mongrels, who, their owners assured me, were the finest hunting dogs in West Africa. I called this untidy ensemble of men and dogs the Bafut Beagles. Although the hunters did not understand the meaning of this title they grew extremely proud of it, and I once heard a hunter, when arguing with a neighbour, proclaim in shrill and indignant tones, 'You no go shout me like dat, ma friend. You no savvay dat I be Bafut Beagle?'

Our hunting method was as follows: we would walk out to some remote hillside or valley, and then choose a thick patch of grass and bushes. At a suitable point we would spread the nets in a half-moon shape; then, with the dogs, we would walk through the undergrowth, driving whatever creatures we found there into the nets. Each dog wore round its neck a little wooden bell, so that when the pack disappeared into the long grass we could still keep a track on their whereabouts by the loud clonking noise from these ornaments. The advantage of this method of hunting was that I was on the spot to handle the creatures from the very moment of capture, and they could be hastily transported back to Bafut and placed in decent cages with the minimum of delay. We transported our captures in bags with special air holes, ringed with brass, let into the sides; for the bigger and tougher creatures the bags were of canvas or hessian, and for the more delicate beasts they were made out of soft cloth. Once in the darkness of the bag the captives generally ceased to struggle, and lay quite quiet until we got them home again; the most frightening part of the process from the animals' point of view was disentangling them from the net, but after a bit of practice we got this down to a fine art, and an animal could be caught, removed from the net, and placed in a bag within the space of two minutes.

The first day that I went out with the Bafut Beagles the hunters turned up so heavily armed one would have thought that we were going out to hunt a lion. Apart from the usual machetes, they were carrying spears and flintlocks. As I did not fancy receiving a backside full of rusty nails and gravel, I insisted, amid much lamentation, that the guns be left behind. The hunters were horrified at my decision.

'Masa,' said one of them plaintively, 'if we go meet bad beef how we go kill um if we go lef' our gun for dis place?'

'If we go meet bad beef we go catch um, no kill um,' I said firmly.

'Eh! Masa go catch bad beef?'

'Na so, my friend. If you fear, you no go come, you hear?'

'Masa, I no de fear,' he said indignantly; 'but if we go meet bad beef and it go kill Masa, de Fon get angry too much.'

'Hush your mouth, my friend,' I said, producing the shotgun. 'I go take my own gun. Den if beef go kill me it no be your palaver, you hear?'

'I hear, sah,' said the hunter.

It was very early morning, and the sun had not yet risen above the encircling mountain ranges. The sky was a very delicate shade of rose pink, trimmed here and there with a lacing of white cloud. The valleys and hills were still blurred and obscured with mist, and the long golden grass at the roadside was bent and heavy with dew. The hunters walked ahead in single file, the pack of dogs scampering in and out of the undergrowth, their bells making a pleasant clonking as they ran. Presently we turned off the road and followed a narrow twisting pathway that led over the hills. Here the mist was thicker, but low-lying. You could not see the lower half of your body, and you got the eerie impression that you were wading waist deep in a smooth and gently undulating lake of foam. The long grass, moist with dew, squeaked across my shoes, and all around me, under the surface of this opaque mist lake, tiny frogs were sharing an amphibian joke with each other in a series of explosive chuckles. Soon the sun rose like a frosted orange above the distant fringe of hills, and as its heat grew stronger the mist started to rise from the ground and coil up to the sky, until it seemed as though we were walking through a forest of pale white trees that twisted and bent, broke and re-formed with amoebic skill as they stretched and spiralled their way upwards. It took us about two hours to reach our destination, the place that the hunters had chosen for our first hunt. It was a deep, wide valley lying between two ridges of hills, curving slightly, like a bow. Along the bottom of this valley a tiny stream made its way between black rocks and golden grass, glinting in the sun like a fine skein of spun glass. The undergrowth in the valley was thick and tangled, shaded here and there by small clumps of shrubs and bushes.

We made our way down into the valley, and there spread about a hundred yards of nets right across it. Then the hunters took the dogs and went to the head of the valley, while I waited near the nets. For half an hour there was silence as they moved slowly towards the net, a silence broken only by the faint sounds of the dogs' bells and an occasional shrill expletive from the hunters when one of them trod on a thorn. I was just beginning to think that we had drawn a blank when the hunters started a great uproar and the dogs began barking furiously. They were still some distance away from the net, and hidden from my view by a small clump of trees.

'Na whatee?' I shouted above the noise.

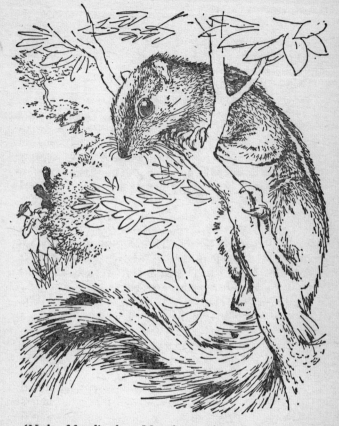

'Na beef for dis place, Masa,' came the answer.

I waited patiently, and presently a panting hunter burst through the trees.

'Masa, you go give me dis small catch-net,' he said, pointing at the smaller nets neatly piled beside the bags.

'Na what kind of beef you done find?' I asked him.

'Na squirrel, sah. 'E done run for up stick.'

I picked up a thick canvas bag, and followed him through the undergrowth until we reached the clump of trees. Here the hunters were grouped, all chattering and arguing as to the best way of catching the quarry, while the dogs leapt and barked round the trunk of a small tree.

'Which side dis beef?' I asked.

'We go catch um one time, Masa.'

'Na fine beef dis, Masa.'

'We go catch um one time, Masa.'

I stepped to the base of the tree and peered up into the foliage; there, perched on a branch some twenty feet above us, was a large and handsome squirrel, of a brindled grey colour with a white stripe along his ribs, and orange paws. His tail was long and not bushy, banded faintly with grey and black. He squatted on the branch, occasionally flipping his tail at us and crying 'Chuck!... chuck!' in a testy sort of manner, as though he was more irritated than alarmed. He watched us with a malevolent eye while we set up the nets in a circle, about ten feet away from the base of the tree. Then we tied up the dogs, and the smallest of the hunters was detailed to climb after the squirrel and drive him down. This latter part of the operation was the hunters' idea; I felt that to try and out-manoeuvre a squirrel in a tree would be impossible, but the hunters insisted that once someone climbed up, the squirrel would come down to the ground. As it turned out they were quite right: no sooner had the hunter reached the upper branches on one side of the tree than the squirrel shot down the trunk on the other side. With incredible cunning he dashed at the one part of the net that had a tear in it, struggled through the hole, and galloped off through the grass, the hunters and myself in hot pursuit, all of us shouting instructions to one another which were completely disregarded. We rounded a clump of bushes to see the squirrel scrambling up the trunk of another small tree.

Once again we spread the nets, and once again the hunter climbed up after the squirrel. This time, however, our quarry was more cunning, for he saw that we were guarding the hole in the net through which he had escaped last time. He ran down the tree-trunk on to the ground, gathered himself into a bunch, and jumped. He sailed through the air and cleared the top of the net by about half an inch; the hunter nearest to him made a wild grab, but missed him, and the squirrel galloped off chuck-chucking indignantly to himself. This time he decided on new evasive tactics, and so instead of climbing up a tree, he dived into a hole at the base of one of them.

Once again we surrounded the tree with nets, and then started to poke long, slender sticks down into the network of tunnel in which he was hiding. This, however, had no effect whatsoever, except to make him chuck a bit faster, so we gave it up. Our next attempt was more successful: we stuffed a handful of smouldering grass into the largest hole, and as the pungent smoke was swept through the various tunnels we could hear the squirrel coughing and sneezing in an angry fashion. At last he could bear it no longer and dashed out of one of the holes, diving head-first into the nets. But even then he had not finished causing trouble, for he bit me and two of the hunters while we were disentangling him, and bit a third hunter while he was being forced into a canvas bag. I hung the bag on the branches of a small bush, and we all sat down to have a much-needed smoke while the squirrel peered at us through the brass-ringed air holes and chattered ferociously, daring us to open the bag and face him.

The Side-striped Ground Squirrels are common enough in the grasslands of West Africa, but I was pleased to have caught this one, as he was the first live specimen I had obtained. As their name implies, these squirrels are almost completely terrestrial in their habits, so it rather surprised me to see the one we had caught taking refuge up in the trees. I discovered later that all the grassland squirrels (most of which *are* terrestrial) made straight for the trees when pursued, and only chose holes in the ground, or hollow logs, as a last resort.

Presently, when we had bound up our wounds, smoked cigarettes, and congratulated each other on our first capture, we moved the big net farther down the valley, to an area where the grass was thick and tangled and almost six feet tall. This was a good place for a special kind of beef, the hunters informed me, though, with understandable caution, they refused to specify what kind. We set up the net, I placed myself at a suitable point half-way along it and inside the curve, so that I could disentangle anything that was caught, and the hunters took the dogs and made their way about a quarter of a mile up the valley. They gave a prolonged yodel to let me know they had started to beat through the long grass, and then silence descended. All I could hear was the whirr and tick of innumerable grasshoppers and locusts around me, and the faint sounds of the dogs' bells. Half an hour passed and nothing happened; I was hemmed in by tall, rustling grass, so thick and interwoven that it was impossible to see through it for more than a couple of feet.

The tiny clearing in which I was sitting shimmered with heat, and I began to feel extremely thirsty; looking round, I noticed something that I had forgotten: a thermos flask of tea which my thoughtful cook had stuck into one of the collecting bags. Thankfully, I got it out, and, squatting down at the edge of the long grass, poured myself a cup. As I was drinking, I noticed the mouth of a dark tunnel in the wall of grass opposite to where I was squatting; it was obviously some creature's private pathway through the forest of grass stalks, and I decided that when I had finished my drink I would investigate it.

I had just poured out my second cup of tea when a terrific uproar broke out to my right, and startlingly near at hand; the hunters were uttering shrill yelps to encourage the dogs, and the dogs were barking furiously. I was just wondering what it was all about when I heard a rustling noise in the grass; I moved closer to the tunnel to try to see what was causing the sound, when quite suddenly the grass parted and a large dark-brown shape hurled itself out of the hole and ran straight into me. I was at a distinct disadvantage: to begin with, I was not expecting the attack, and secondly, I was squatting on my heels, clasping a thermos flask in one hand and a cup of tea in the other. The animal, which, to my startled eyes, seemed to be twice the size of a beaver, landed amidships, and I went flat on my back, the creature on my stomach, and the thermos flask pouring a stream of scalding tea into my lap with deadly accuracy. Both the creature and I seemed equally astonished, and our shrill squeals of fright were almost identical. My hands were full, so I could do nothing more than make a wild grab at him with my arms, but he bounded off me like a rubber ball and scuttled away through the grass. A portion of the net started to jerk and quiver, and despairing squeals were wafted to me, so I presumed that he must have run straight into the net. Shouting for the hunters, I struggled through the long grass towards the spot where the net was moving.

Our quarry had entangled himself very thoroughly, and he lay hunched up in the net, quivering and snorting, and occasionally making ineffectual attempts to bite through the mesh. Peering at it, I could see we had caught a very large Cane Rat, a creature known to the Africans as a Cutting-grass, a name which describes its habits very well, for with its large and well-developed incisors the Cutting-grass goes through the grass-fields – and the farmlands – like a mowing machine. It measured about two and a half feet in length, and was covered with a coarse brownish fur. It had a chubby, rather beaver-like face, small ears set close to the head, a thick naked tail, and large naked feet. It seemed so scared of my presence that I did not approach it until the hunters arrived, for fear it would break out of the net. It lay there quivering violently, and occasionally giving little jerks and leaps into the air, accompanying them with a despairing squeal. At the time, this action worried me quite a lot, for it looked as though the creature was in the last stages of a heart attack. It was only later when I grew to know these animals better, that I discovered they greeted any unusual experience with this display of hysteria, in the hope, I suppose, of frightening or confusing the enemy. In reality, Cane Rats are not very timid animals and would not hesitate to bury their large incisors in the back of your hand if you tried to take liberties with them. I kept a discreet distance until the hunters joined me; then we went forward and removed the rat from the net.

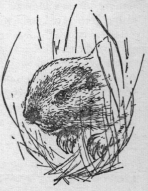

While we were manoeuvring him from the net into a stout

bag, he suddenly jumped violently in my hands; to my surprise, as I tightened my grip on him, a large quantity of his fur came away in my fingers. When we had him safely in the bag, I sat down and examined the hair that my clutch had removed from his fat body: it was fairly long and quite thick, more like a coarse bristle; it is apparently planted so loosely in the skin that it comes away in handfuls at the slightest pull. Once it has come away, the hair takes a remarkably long time to grow again, and, as bald Cane Rats are not exactly beautiful, one had to handle them with extreme care.

After we had captured the Cane Rat we made our way slowly up the valley, spreading the net at intervals and beating likely-looking patches of undergrowth. When it was obvious that the valley would yield no more specimens, we rolled up the nets and made our way towards a large hill about half a mile away. This hill was so beautifully formed that it might well have been a barrow, the grave of some giant who had prowled the grassland in days gone by; on the very top was a cluster of boulders, each the size of a house, rearing themselves up like a monument. Growing in the narrow crevices and gullies between these rocks were a number of tiny trees, their trunks twisted and crumpled by the winds, each bearing a small cluster of bright golden fruit. In the long grass round the base of the trunks grew several purple and yellow orchids, and in places the great rocks were covered with a thick mat of climbing plant, a kind of convolvulus, from which dangled the ivory-coloured, trumpet-shaped flowers. The great pile of rocks, the bright flowers and the shaggy and misshapen trees formed a wonderful picture against the smouldering blue of the afternoon sky.

We climbed up into the shade of these rocks and squatted in the long grass to have our meal. The mountain grassland spread away from us in all directions, its multitude of colours shimmering and changing with the wind. The hill-crests were pale gold changing to white, while the valleys were pale greeny-blue, darker in places where a pompous cumulus cloud swept over, trailing a purple shadow in its wake. Directly ahead of us lay a long range of delicately sculptured hills whose base was almost hidden in a litter of great boulders and small trees. The hills were so smoothly and beautifully formed, and clad in grass which showed such a bewildering variety of greens, golds, purples, and whites, that they looked like a great rambling wave rearing up to break over the puny barrier of rocks and shrubs below. The peace and silence of these heights was remarkable; nearly all sounds were created by the wind, and it was busy moving here and there, making each object produce its own song. It combed the grass and brought forth a soft, lisping rustle; it squeezed and wriggled between the cracks and joints of the rocks above us and made owl-like moans and sudden hoots of mirth; it pushed and wrestled with the tough little trees, making them creak and groan, and making their leaves flutter and purr like kittens. Yet all these small sounds seemed to enhance rather than destroy the silence of the grassland.

Suddenly the silence was shattered by a terrific uproar that broke out behind the massive pile of rocks. Working my way round there, I found the hunters and dogs in a group at the base of a giant rock. Three of the hunters were arguing vigorously with each other, while the fourth was dancing about, yelping with pain and scattering large quantities of blood from a wound in his hand, with the excited dogs leaping and barking frenziedly around him.

'Na whatee dis palaver?' I asked.

All four hunters turned on me and offered their separate descriptions of the event, their voices becoming louder and louder as they tried to shout each other down.

'Why you all de shout? How I go hear if you all go talk together like women, eh?' I said.

Having thus produced silence, I pointed at the bloodstained hunter.

'Now, how you done get dis wound, ma friend?'

'Masa, beef done chop me.'

'Beef? What kind of beef?'

'Eh! Masa, I no savvay. 'E de bite *too much*, sah.'

I examined his hand and found that a chunk the size of a shilling had been neatly removed from the palm. I rendered

primitive first-aid, and then went into the matter of the animal
that had bitten him.

'Which side dis beef?'

''E dere dere for dat hole, sah,' said the wounded one,
pointing at a cleft in the base of a large rock.

'You no savvay what kind of beef?'

'No, sah,' he said aggrievedly, 'I no see um. I go come for
dis place an' I see dat hole. I tink sometime dere go be beef
for inside, so I done put ma hand for dere. Den dis beef 'e
done chop me.'

'Whah! Dis man no get fear,' I said, turning to the other
hunters, 'he no go look de hole first. He done put his hand for
inside and beef done chop him.'

The other hunters giggled. I turned to the wounded man
again.

'Ma friend, you done put your hand for dis hole, eh? Now,
sometimes you go find snake for dis kind of place, no be so?
If snake done chop you what you go do?'

'I no savvay, Masa,' he said, grinning.

'I no want dead hunter man, ma friend, so you no go do
dis sort of foolish thing again, you hear?'

'I hear, sah.'

'All right. Now we go look dis beef that done chop you.'

Taking a torch from the collecting bag I crouched down by
the hole and peered up it. In the torch beam a pair of small
eyes glowed ruby red, and then a little, pointed, ginger-
coloured face appeared round them, uttered a shrill, snarling
screech, and disappeared into the gloom at the back of the hole.

'Ah!' said one of the hunters who had heard the noise,
'dis na bush dog. Dis beef 'e fierce too much, sah.'

Unfortunately, the pidgin English term 'bush dog' is used
indiscriminately to describe a great variety of small mammals,
few of which are even remotely related to dogs, so the hunter's
remark left me none the wiser as to what sort of an animal it
was. After some argument, we decided that the best way to get
the beast to show itself was to light a fire outside the hole, and
then blow smoke into it by fanning with a bunch of leaves.
This we proceeded to do, having first hung a small net over

the mouth of the hole. The first whiff of smoke had hardly drifted in amongst the rocks when the beast shot out of the hole and into the net with such force that it was torn from its moorings, and the animal rolled down the slope into the long grass, carrying the net with him. The dogs scrambled after him, barking uproariously with excitement, and we followed close on their heels, yelling threats as to what punishment they would receive if they harmed the quarry. However, the beast hardly needed our help, for he was perfectly capable of looking after himself, as we soon found out.

He shook himself free of the folds of netting, and stood up on his hind legs, revealing himself as a slim ginger mongoose, about the size of a stoat. He stood there, swaying slightly from side to side, his mouth wide open, uttering the shrillest and most ear-piercing shrieks I have ever heard from an animal of that size. The dogs pulled up short and surveyed him in consternation as he swayed and shrieked before them; one, slightly braver than the rest, moved forward gingerly and sniffed at this strange creature. This was obviously what the mongoose had been waiting for; he dropped flat in the grass and slid forward like a snake, disappearing among the long grass stalks, and then suddenly reappearing in between the feet of our noble pack, where he proceeded to whirl round like a top, biting at every paw and leg in sight, and keeping up an incessant yarring scream as he did so. The dogs did their best to avoid his jaws, but they were at a disadvantage, for the long grass hid his approach, and all they could do was leap wildly in the air. Then, suddenly, their courage failed them, and they all turned tail and fled up the hill again, leaving the mongoose standing on his hind legs in the field of battle, panting slightly, but still able to screech taunts at their retreating tails.

The pack having thus been vanquished, it was left to us to try to capture this fierce, if diminutive, adversary. This we accomplished more easily than I had thought possible: I attracted his attention, and then got him to attack a canvas collecting bag, and while he was busily engaged in biting this, one of the hunters crept round behind him and threw a net over him. During the time we were disentangling the mongoose from

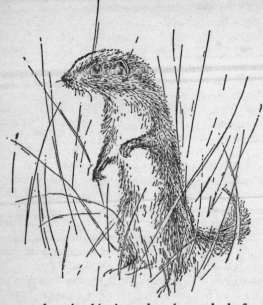

the net and getting him into a bag, he nearly deafened us with
his screams of rage, and he kept up this ghastly noise all the
way home, though mercifully it was slightly muffled by the
thick canvas. He did not stop until, on reaching Bafut, I tipped
him into a large cage and threw in a gory chicken's head. He
settled down to eat this in a very philosophical manner, and
soon finished it. After that he remained silent, except when he
caught sight of anyone, and then he would rush to the bars and
start to scream abuse at them. It became so nerve-racking in
the end that I was forced to cover the front of his cage with a
bit of sacking until he had become more used to human com-
pany. Three days later I heard those familiar screeches echoing
down the road, and long before the native hunter appeared in
sight I knew that another Dwarf Mongoose was being brought
in. I was pleased to find that this second one was a young
female, so I put her in with the one we had already captured.
This was rather unwise of me, for they took to screaming in

chorus, each trying to outdo the other, until the noise was as soothing as a knife drawn sideways across a plate, magnified several thousand times.

On arrival back at Bafut after my first day out with the Beagles, I received a note from the Fon asking me to go over to his house for a drink and to give him any hunting news there might be, so when I had eaten and changed I set off across the great courtyard and presently came to the Fon's little villa. He was seated on the veranda, holding a bottle of gin up to the light to see what the contents were.

'Ah, ma friend!' he said, 'you done come? You done have good hunting for bush?'

'Yes,' I said, taking the chair he offered, 'hunter man for Bafut savvay catch fine beef. We done catch three beef.'

'Foine, foine,' said the Fon, pouring out five fingers of gin into a glass and handing it to me. 'You go stay here small time you go get plenty beef. I go tell all ma peoples.'

'Na so. I think Bafut people savvay catch beef pass all people for Cameroons.'

'Na true, na true,' said the Fon delightedly; 'you speak true, ma friend.'

We raised our glasses, chinked them together, beamed at one another, and then drank deeply. The Fon filled up the glasses again, and then sent one of his numerous retinue in search of a fresh bottle. By the time we had worked our way through most of this bottle we had mellowed considerably, and the Fon turned to me:

'You like musica?' he inquired.

'Yes, too much,' I said, truthfully, for I had heard that the Fon possessed a band of more than usual skill.

'Good! We go have some musica,' he said, and issued a terse command to one of his servants.

Presently the band filed into the compound below the veranda, and to my surprise it consisted of about twenty of the Fon's wives, all naked except for meagre loin-cloths. They were armed with a tremendous variety of drums, ranging from one the size of a small saucepan to the great deep-bellied specimens that required two people to carry them; there were also wooden and bamboo flutes that had a curious sweetness of tone, and large bamboo boxes filled with dried maize that gave forth a wonderful rustling rattle when shaken. But the most curious instrument in the band was a wooden pipe about four feet long. This was held upright, one end resting on the ground, and blown into in a special way, producing a deep, vibrating noise that was quite astonishing, for it was the sort of sound you would expect to come only from a lavatory with exceptional acoustics.

The band began to play, and soon various members of the Fon's household started to dance in the compound. The dance consisted of a sort of cross between folk dancing and ballroom dancing. The couples, clasping each other, would gyrate slowly round and round, their feet performing tiny and complicated steps, while their bodies wiggled and swayed in a way that no Palais de Danse would have allowed. Occasionally, a couple would break apart and each twirl off on their own for a time, doing their own swaying steps to the music, completely absorbed. The flutes twittered and squeaked, the drums galloped and shuddered, the rattles crashed and rustled with the monotonous regularity of waves on a shingle beach, and steadily, behind this frenzy of sound, you could hear the tuba-like instruments' cry, a gigantic catharsis every few seconds with the constancy of a heartbeat.

'You like my musica?' shouted the Fon.

'Yes, na very fine,' I roared back.

'You get dis kind of musica for your country?'

'No,' I said with genuine regret, 'we no get um.'

The Fon filled my glass again.

'Soon, when my people bring grass, we go have plenty musica, plenty dancing, eh? We go have happy time, we go be happy too much, no be so?'

'Yes, na so. We go have happy time.'

Outside in the compound the band played on, and the steady roll and thud of the drums seemed to drift up into the dark sky and make even the stars shiver and dance to their rhythm.

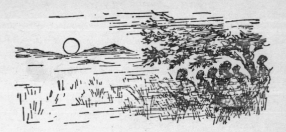

CHAPTER THREE

The Squirrel That Booms

THERE were two species of the grassland fauna that I was very anxious to obtain during my stay in Bafut; one was the Rock Hyrax, and the other was Stanger's Squirrel. To get them I had to undertake two hunts in very different types of country, and they remain in my mind more vividly than almost all the other hunting experiences I had in the grasslands.

The first of these hunts was after the squirrel, and it was chiefly remarkable because for once I was able to plan a campaign in advance and carry it through successfully without any last-minute, unforeseen hitches. Stanger's squirrel is a reasonably common animal in the Cameroons, but previously I had hunted for it in the deep forest in the Mamfe basin. In this sort of country it spent its time in the top branches of the higher trees (feeding on the rich banquet of fruit growing in those sunny heights) and rarely coming down to ground level. This made its capture almost impossible. However, I had since learnt that in the grassland the squirrel frequented the small patches of forest on river-banks, and spent quite a large part of its time on the ground, foraging in the grass for food. This, I felt, would give one a better chance of capturing it. When I had shown a picture of the squirrel to the Bafut Beagles, they identified it immediately, and vociferously maintained that they knew where it was to be found. Questioning them, I discovered that they knew the habits of the creature quite well, for they had hunted it often.

Apparently the squirrels lived in a small patch of mountain forest, but in the very early morning or in the evening they came down from the trees and ventured into the grassland to feed. Then, said the Bafut Beagles, was the time to catch them. What, I asked, did this beef do during the night?

'Ah! Masa, you no fit catch um for night time,' came the reply; 'dis beef 'e de sleep for up dat big stick where no man fit pass. But for evening time, or early-early morning time we fit catch um.'

'Right,' I said, 'we go catch um for early-early morning time.'

We left Bafut at one o'clock in the morning, and after a long and tedious walk over hills, through valleys and grassfields, we reached our destination an hour before dawn. It was a small plateau that lay half-way up a steep mountain-side. The area was comparatively flat, and across it tinkled a wide and shallow stream, along the sides of which grew a thick but narrow strip of forest. Crouching in the lee of a big rock, peering into the gloom and wiping the dew from our faces, we spied out the land and made our plans. The idea was to erect two or three strips of net in the long grass about five hundred yards away from the edge of the trees. This we had to do immediately, before it got so light that the squirrels could see us.

Erecting nets in long grass up to your waist, when it is sodden with dew, is not a soothing pastime, and we were glad when the last one had been tied in place. Then we cautiously approached the forest, and crawled into hiding beneath a large bush. Here we squatted, trying to keep our teeth from chattering, not able to smoke or talk or move, watching the eastern sky grow paler as the darkness of the night was drained out of it. Slowly it turned to a pale opalescent grey, then it flushed to pink, and then, as the sun rose above the horizon, it turned suddenly and blindingly to a brilliant kingfisher blue. This pure and delicate light showed the mountains around us covered in low-lying mist; as the sun rose higher, the mist started to move and slide on the ridges and pour down the hillsides to fill the valleys. For one brief instant we had seen the grasslands quiet and asleep under the blanket of mist; now it seemed as though the mountains were awakening, yawning and stretching under the white coverlet, pushing it aside in some places, gathering it more tightly in others, hoisting itself, dew-misted and sleepy, from the depths of its white bedclothes. On many occasions later I watched this awakening of the mountains, and I never wearied of the sight. Considering that the same thing has been happening each morning since the ancient mountains came into being, it is astonishing how fresh and new the sight appears each time you witness it. Never does it become dull and mechanical; it is always different: sometimes the mist in rising shaped itself into strange animal shapes – dragons, phoenix, wyvern, and milk-white unicorns – sometimes it would form itself into strange, drifting strands of seaweed, trees, or great tumbling bushes of white flowers; occasionally, if there was a breeze to help it, it would startle you by assuming the most severe and complicated geometrical shapes, while all the time, underneath it, in tantalizing glimpses as it shifted, you could see the mountains gleaming in a range of soft colours so delicate and ethereal that it was impossible to put a name to them.

I decided as I squatted there, peering between the branches of the bush we sheltered under, watching the mountains waken, that it was worth feeling tired, cold, and hungry, worth being drenched with dew and suffering cramps, in order to see such a sight. My meditations were interrupted by a loud and aggressive 'Chuck ... chuck!' from the trees above us, and one of the hunters gripped my arm and looked at me with glowing eyes. He leant forward slowly and whispered in my ear:

'Masa, dis na de beef Masa want. We go sit softly softly 'e go come down for ground small time.'

I wiped the dew from my face and peered out at the grass-field where we had set the nets. Presently we heard other chucking noises from deeper in the forest as more of the squirrels awoke and glanced at the day with suspicious eyes. We waited for what seemed a long time, and then I suddenly saw something moving in the grassfield between us and the nets: a curious object that at first sight looked like an elongated black-and-white-striped balloon, appearing now and then

47

above the long grass. In that mist-blurred morning haze I could not make out what this strange object could be, so I attracted the hunters' attention and pointed to it silently.

'Dis na de beef, Masa,' said one.

''E done go for ground, 'e done go for ground,' said the other gleefully.

'Na whatee dat ting?' I whispered, for I could not reconcile that strange balloon-like object with any part of a squirrel's anatomy.

'Dis ting na 'e tail, sah,' explained a hunter, and, so that I should be left in no doubt, 'dat ting 'e get for 'e larse.'

Like all tricks, once it had been explained, it became obvious. I could see quite clearly that the black-and-white-striped object *was* a squirrel's tail, and I wondered why on earth I had thought that it resembled a balloon. Presently the one tail was joined by others, and as the mist lifted and cleared we could see the squirrels themselves.

There were eight of them hopping out into the grassfield. They were large and rather bulky animals, with heavy heads, but the largest and most flamboyant parts of their anatomies were their tails. They hopped cautiously from tussock to tussock, pausing to sit up on their hind legs and sniff carefully in the direction they were travelling. Then they would get down and hop forward a few more feet, flipping their tails as they moved. Sometimes they would crouch perfectly still for a few seconds, their tails laid carefully over their backs, the bushy ends hanging down and almost obscuring their faces. The ones in the grassfield were silent, but in the trees behind us we could still hear an occasional suspicious 'chuck' from those that had not yet plucked up the courage to descend. I decided that eight would be quite enough for us to try to catch, so I signalled the hunters and we rose from our hide-out. We spread out in a line through the trees, and then the hunters paused and waited for the signal to advance.

The squirrels were now about a hundred and fifty yards from the forest's edge, and I decided that this was far enough for our purposes. I waved my hand, and then we walked out from the shelter of the trees into the long grass. The squirrels

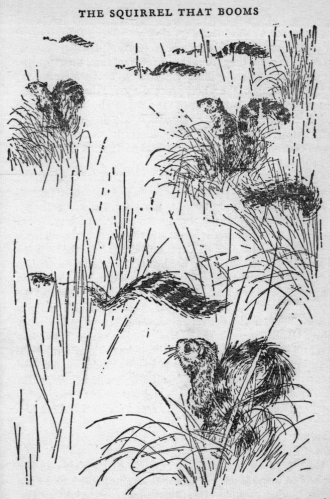

in the forest gave loud chucks of alarm, and the squirrels in the grassfield sat up on their hind legs to see what was the matter. They saw us and all froze instantly; then, as we moved slowly forward, they hopped off into the grass, farther and farther from the trees. I do not think they could quite make out what we were, for we advanced very slowly and with the minimum of movement. They felt we were something hostile, but they were not certain; they would run a few yards and then stop and sit up to survey us, sniffing vigorously. This was really the most tricky part of the whole proceeding, for the animals were not yet within the half circle of the nets, and by breaking away to left or right they could easily escape into the grassfields. We drifted towards them cautiously, the only sounds being the swish of our feet in the grass and faint and frantic chucks from the forest behind us.

Quite suddenly one squirrel more quick-witted than the rest realized what was happening. He could not see the nets ahead, for they were hidden in the long grass and well camouflaged, but he saw that as we advanced we were driving him farther and farther away from the forest and the safety of the tall trees. He gave a loud chuck of alarm and dashed off through the grass, his long tail streaming out behind him, and then suddenly twisted to the left and galloped through the grass away from the nets. His one ambition was to get round us and back to the trees. The rest of the squirrels sat up and watched him nervously, and I realized that unless something was done they would all pluck up courage and follow his example. I had planned to wait until they were well within the circle of nets before charging down on them and causing a panic that would send them scuttling into the mesh, but it now became obvious that we should have to take a chance and stampede them. I raised my hand, and the hunters and I surged forward, yelling and hooting, waving our arms and trying to appear as fearsome as possible. For a split second the squirrels watched us without movement; then they fled.

Four of them followed the example of the first one and dashed off at right angles, thus avoiding both the hunters and the nets; the remaining three, however, ran straight for our trap, and, as we dashed towards the scene we could see the top of the net jerking – a certain indication that they had got themselves entangled. Sure enough, we found them firmly entwined, glaring out at us and giving vent to the loudest and most awesome gurking noises I have heard from a squirrel. It was a completely different sound from the loud chuck that they had been making: it was fearsome and full of warning – a cross between a snore and a snarl. They kept this up while we were unwinding them, giving savage bites at our hands with their great orange incisors. When we had at last got them into canvas bags we had to hang the bags on the end of a stick to carry them, for, unlike the other grassland squirrels, who lay quietly when they were put in the gloom of a bag, these creatures seemed quite willing to continue the fight, and the slightest touch on the outside of the bag would be greeted by a furious attack and a rapid series of gurks.

The squirrels in the forest were thoroughly alarmed, and the trees echoed to the sound of frantic chuckings. Now that they had realized how dangerous we were it was useless to try to attempt another capture, so we had to be content with the three we had caught; we packed up our nets and other equipment and made our way back to Bafut. Once there I placed my precious squirrels in three solid, tin-lined cages, filled their plates with food, and left them severely alone until they should have recovered from the indignity of capture. As soon as they were left alone they ventured out of the darkness of their bedrooms and demolished the pile of succulent fruits with which I had provided them, upset their water-pots, tested the tin lining of the cages to see if they could be gnawed through, and, finding that this was impossible, retired to their bedrooms again and slept. Seen at close quarters they were quite handsome beasts, with pale yellow bellies and cheeks, russet-red backs, and great banded tails. The effect was somewhat spoilt by their heads, which were large and rather horse-like, with tiny ears set close to the skull, and protuberant teeth.

I had read somewhere that these squirrels climb to the top branches of the forest trees in the early morning and utter the most powerful and astonishing cries: deep rolling sounds that were like the last notes of a giant gong being struck. I was interested to hear this cry, but I thought it unlikely that they would produce it in captivity. However, the morning after the capture I was awakened at about five-thirty by a peculiar noise; the collection was on the veranda outside my window, and when I sat up in bed I decided that the noise was coming from one of the cages, but I could not tell from which. I put on my dressing-gown and crept out of the door. I waited patiently in the dim light, chilly and half awake, for a repetition of the sound. It came again in a few minutes, and I could definitely trace it to the squirrels' cage. The noise is extremely difficult to describe: it started like a groan, and as it got louder it took on a throbbing, vibrating note, the sort of thrumming you hear from telegraph poles – the sound seemed to blur and waver, like a gong hit very softly, rising to a crescendo and then dying away. The squirrels were obviously being rather half-hearted about their attempt; in the forest they would have put much more force into it, and then I should imagine it would be a weird and fascinating cry to hear, drifting through the misty branches.

That evening the Fon appeared, as usual, to find out what success the day had brought, and to present me with a calabash of fresh palm wine. With great pride I showed him the squirrels, and described the capture in detail for him. He was intrigued to know exactly where we had caught them, and, as I did not really know the locality, I had to go and call one of the hunters – who was merry-making in the kitchen – to explain to him. He stood in front of the Fon, answering his questions through cupped hands. It took quite a long time for the hunter to do this, for the country we had been in was uninhabited, so he could only describe our route by reference to various landmarks in the shape of rocks, trees, and curiously shaped hills. At last the Fon started to nod vigorously, and then sat for a few minutes in thought. Then he spoke to the hunter rapidly, making wide gestures with his long arms, while the hunter nodded and bowed. At length the Fon turned to me, smiling benignly, and carelessly, almost absent-mindedly, holding out his empty glass.

'I done tell dis man,' he explained, watching me fill the glass with an apparently uninterested eye, ''e go take you for some special place for mountain. For dis place you get some special kind of beef.'

'What kind of beef?' I asked.

'Beef,' said the Fon vaguely, gesturing with his half-empty glass, 'special kind of beef. You no get um yet.'

'Na bad beef dis?' I suggested.

The Fon put his glass on the table and spread out his enormous hands.

'Na so big,' he said, 'no be bad bad beef, but 'e bite too much. 'E go live for dat big big rock, 'e go go for under. Sometime 'e de hollar too much, 'e go Wheeeeeeeee!!!'

I sat and puzzled over the creature, while the Fon watched me hopefully.

''E look same same for Cutting-grass, but 'e no get tail for 'e larse,' he said at last, helpfully.

Light suddenly dawned, and I went in search of a book; I found the picture I wanted, and showed it to the Fon.

'Dis na de beef?' I asked.

'Ah! Na so,' said the Fon delightedly, stroking the portrait of the rock hyrax with his long fingers; 'dis na de beef. How you de call um?'

'Rock hyrax.'

'Rooke hyrix?'

'Yes. How you de call um for Bafut?'

'Here we call um N'eer.'

I wrote the name down on the list of local names I was compiling, and then refilled the Fon's glass. He was still gazing in a trance at the engraving of the hyrax, tracing its outline with one slender finger.

'Wha!' he said at length in a wistful voice, 'na fine chop dis beef. You go cook um with coco yam ...'

His voice died away and he licked his lips reminiscently.

The hunter fixed me with his eye, and shuffled his feet as an indication that he wanted to speak.

'Yes, na whatee?'

'Masa want to go for dis place de Fon de talk?'

'Yes. We go go to-morrow for morning time.'

'Yes, sah. For catch dis beef Masa go need plenty people. Dis beef fit run too much, sah.'

'All right, you go tell all my boys dey go for bush to-morrow.'

'Yes, sah.'

He stood and shuffled his feet again.

'Whatee?'

'Masa go want me again?'

'No, my friend. Go back for kitchen and drink your wine.'

'Tank you, sah,' he said, grinning, and disappeared into the gloom of the veranda.

Presently the Fon rose to go, and I walked with him as far as the road. As we paused at the edge of the compound he turned and smiled down at me from his great height.

'I be ole man,' he said; 'I de tire too much. If I no be ole man I go come with you for bush to-morrow.'

'You lie, my friend. You no be ole man. You done get power too much. You get plenty power, power pass all dis picken hunter man.'

He chuckled, and then sighed.

'No, my friend, you no speak true. My time done pass. I de tire too much. I get plenty wife, and dey de tire me too much. I get palaver with dis man, with dat man, an' it de tire me too much. Bafut na big place, plenty people. If you get plenty people you get plenty palaver.'

'Na so, I savvay you get plenty work.'

'True,' he said, and then added, his eyes twinkling wickedly, 'sometimes I get palaver with the D.O., an' dat de tire me most of all.'

He shook my hand, and I could hear him chuckling as he walked off across the courtyard.

The next morning we set off on our hyrax hunt – myself, the four Bafut Beagles, and five of the household staff. For the first two or three miles we walked through the cultivated areas and the small farms. On the gently sloping hills fields had been dug, and the rich red earth shone in the early morning sunshine. In some of the fields the crops were already planted and ripe, the feathery bushes of cassava or the row of maize, each golden head with its blond tassel of silken thread waving in the breeze. In other fields the women were working, stripped to the waist, wielding short-handled, broad-bladed hoes. Some of them had tiny babies strapped to their backs, and they seemed as unaware of these encumbrances as a hunchback would be of his hump. Most of the older ones were smoking long black pipes, and the rank grey smoke swirled up into their faces as they bent over the ground. It was mostly the younger women who were doing the harder work of hoeing, and their lithe, glistening bodies moved rhythmically in the sun as they raised the heavy and clumsy implements high above their heads and then brought them sweeping down. Each time the blade buried itself in the red earth the owner would give a loud grunt.

As we walked through the fields among them they talked with us in their shrill voices, made jokes, and laughed uproariously, all without pausing in their work, and without losing its rhythm. The grunts that interspersed their remarks gave a curious sound to the conversation.

'Morning, Masa ... ugh! ... which side you go? ... ugh!'

'Masa go go for bush ... ugh! ... no be so, Masa? ... ugh!'

'Masa go catch plenty beef ... ugh! ... Masa get power ... ugh!'

'Walker strong, Masa ... ugh! ... catch beef *plenty* ... ugh!'

Long after we had left the fields and were scrambling up the golden slopes of the foothills we could hear them chattering and laughing and the steady thump of the hoes striking home.

When we reached the crest of the highest range of hills that surrounded Bafut the hunters pointed out our destination: a range of mountains, purple and misty, that seemed an enormous distance away. The household staff gave gasps and moans of dismay and astonishment that I should want them to walk so far, and Jacob, the cook, said that he did not think he would be able to manage it, as he had unfortunately picked up a thorn in his foot. Examination proved that there was no thorn in his foot, but a small stone in his shoe. The discovery and removal of the stone left him moody and disgruntled, and he lagged behind, talking to himself in a ferocious undertone. To my surprise, the distance was deceptive, and within three hours we were walking through a long winding valley at the end of which the mountains reared up in a wall of glittering gold and green. As we toiled up the slope through the waist-high grass, the hunters explained to me what the plan of campaign was to be. Apparently we had to round one of the smooth buttresses of the mountain range, and in between this projection and the next lay a long valley that thrust its way into the heart of the mountains. The sides of this valley were composed of almost sheer cliffs, at the base of which were the rocks where hyrax lived.

We scrambled round the great elbow of mountain, and there lay the valley before us, quiet and remote and filled with sparkling sunlight that lit the gaunt cliffs on each side – two long, crumpled curtains of rock flushed to pink and grey, patched with golden sunlight and soft blue shadows. Piled at the base of these cliffs were the legacies of many past cliff falls and landslides, a jumble of boulders of all shapes and sizes, some scattered about the curving floor of the valley, some piled up into tall, tottering chimneys. Over and around these rocks grew a rippling green rug of short undergrowth, long grass, hunched and crafty looking trees, small orchids and tall lilies, and a thick, strangling web of convolvulus with yellow, cream, and pink flowers. Scattered along the cliff faces were a series of cave mouths, dark and mysterious, some mere narrow clefts in the rock, others the size of a cathedral door. Down the centre of the valley ran a boisterous baby stream that wiggled joyfully in and out of the rocks, and leapt impatiently in lacy waterfalls from one level to the next as it hurried down the slope.

We paused at the head of the valley for a rest and a smoke, and I examined the rocks ahead with my field-glasses for any signs of life. But the valley seemed lifeless and deserted; the only sounds were the self-important and rather ridiculous tinkle of the diminutive stream, and the wind and the grass moving together with a stealthy sibilant whisper. High overhead a small hawk appeared against the delicate blue sky, paused for an instant, and swept out of view behind the jagged edge of the cliff. Jacob stood and surveyed the valley with a sour and gloomy expression on his pudgy countenance.

'Na whatee, Jacob?' I asked innocently; 'you see beef?'

'No, sah,' he said, glowering at his feet.

'You no like dis place?'

'No, sah, I no like um.'

'Why?'

'Na bad place dis, sah.'

'Why na bad place?'

'Eh! Sometime for dis kind of place you get bad juju, Masa.'

I looked at the Bafut Beagles, who were lying in the grass.

'You get juju for dis place?' I asked them.

'No, sah, atall,' they said unanimously.

'You see,' I said to Jacob, 'dere no be juju for here, so you no go fear, you hear?'

'Yes, sah,' said Jacob with complete lack of conviction.

'And if you go catch dis beef for me I go give you fine dash,' I went on.

Jacob brightened visibly. 'Masa go give us dash same same for hunter man?' he asked hopefully.

'Na so.'

He sighed and scratched his stomach thoughtfully.

'You still think dere be juju for dis place?'

'Eh!' he said, shrugging, 'sometimes I done make mistake.'

'Ah, Jacob! If Masa go give you dash you go kill your own Mammy,' said one of the Bafut Beagles, chuckling, for Jacob's preoccupation with money was well known in Bafut.

'Wha',' said Jacob angrily, 'an' you no love money, eh? Why you go come for bush with Masa if you no love money, eh?'

'Na my job,' said the hunter, and added by way of explanation, 'I be Beagle.'

Before Jacob could think up a suitable retort to this, one of the other hunters held up his hand.

'Listen, Masa!' he said excitedly.

We all fell silent, and then from the valley ahead a strange cry drifted down to us; it started as a series of short, tremulous whistles, delivered at intervals, and then suddenly turned into a prolonged hoot which echoed weirdly from the rocky walls of the valley.

'Na N'eer dis, Masa,' the Beagles whispered. ''E de hollar for dat big rock dere.'

I trained my field-glasses on the big huddle of rocks they indicated, but it was some seconds before I saw the hyrax. He was squatting on a ledge of rock, surveying the valley with a haughty expression on his face. He was about the size of a large rabbit, but with short, thick legs and a rather blunt, lion-like face. His ears were small and neat, and he appeared to have no tail at all. Presently, as I watched, he turned on the narrow ledge and ran to the top of the rock, paused for a moment to judge the distance, and then leapt lightly to the next pile of boulders and disappeared into a tangle of convolvulus that obviously masked a hole of some sort. I lowered the glasses and looked at the Bafut Beagles.

'Well?' I asked, 'how we go catch dis beef?'

They had a rapid exchange of ideas in their own language, then one of them turned to me.

'Masa,' he said, screwing up his face and scratching his head, 'dis beef 'e cleaver too much. We no fit catch him with net, and 'e fit run pass man.'

'Well, my friend, how we go do?'

'We go find hole for rock, sah, and we go make fire with plenty smoke; we go put net for de hole, an' when de beef run, so we go catch um.'

'All right,' I said; 'come, we go start.'

We started off up the valley, Jacob leading the way with a look of grim determination on his face. We struggled through the thick web of short undergrowth until we reached the first tottering pile of boulders, and there we spread out like terriers, and scrambled and crawled our way round, peering into every crevice to see if it was inhabited. It was Jacob, strangely enough, who first struck lucky; he raised a sweaty and glowing face from the tangle of undergrowth and called to me.

'Masa, I done find hole. 'E get beef for inside,' he said excitedly.

We crowded round the hole and listened. Sure enough, we could hear something stirring inside: faint scrabbling sounds were wafted to us. Rapidly we laid a fire of dried grass in the entrance to the hole, and when it was well alight we covered it with green leaves, which produced a column of thick and

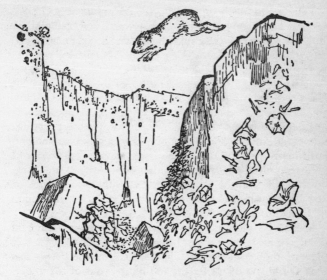

pungent smoke. We hung a net over the hole, and then fanned the smoke into the depths of the rock with the aid of large bunches of leaves. Blown by our vigorous fanning, the smoke rolled and tumbled up the tunnel into the darkness, and then suddenly things began to happen with bewildering rapidity. Two baby hyrax, each the size of a large guinea-pig, shot out into the bushes with it tangled round them. Close on their heels came the mother, a corpulent beast in a towering rage. She raced out of the hole and leapt at the nearest person, who happened to be one of the Beagles; she moved so rapidly that he had not time to get out of her way, and she fastened her teeth in his ankle and hung on like a bulldog, giving loud and terrifying 'Weeeeeeeee!' noises through her nose. The Beagle fell backwards into a great blanket of convolvulus, kicking out wildly with his legs, and uttering loud cries of pain.

The other Beagles were busy trying to disentangle the baby hyrax from the net and were finding it a whole-time job. The household staff had fled at the appearance of the irate mother, so it was left to Jacob and me to go to the rescue of the Beagle who was lashing about in the undergrowth, screaming at the top of his voice. Before I could do anything sensible, however, Jacob came into his own. For once his brain actually caught up with the rapidity of events. His action was not, I fear, the result of any sympathetic consideration for the sufferings of his black brother, but prompted rather by the thought that unless something was done quickly the female hyrax might escape, in which case he would get no money for her. He leapt past me, with extraordinary speed for one normally so somnolent, clutching in his hand one of the larger canvas bags. Before I could stop him he had grabbed the unfortunate Beagle's leg and stuffed it into the bag, together with the hyrax. Then he drew the mouth of the bag tight with a smile of satisfaction and turned to me.

'Masa!' he said, raising his voice above the indignant screams of his countryman, 'I done catch um!'

His triumph, however, was short-lived, for the Beagle had come to the end of his tether, and he rose out of the undergrowth and hit Jacob hard on the back of his woolly head. Jacob gave a roar of anguish and rolled backwards down the slope, while the Beagle rose to his feet and made desperate efforts to rid his foot of the hyrax-infested bag. I regret to admit that I could do nothing more sensible than sit down on a rock and laugh until the tears ran down my face. Jacob also rose to his feet, uttering loud threats, and saw the Beagle trying to remove the bag.

'Arrrr!' he yelled, leaping up the slope; 'stupid man, de beef go run.'

He clasped the Beagle in his arms and they both fell backwards into the undergrowth. By now the other Beagles had successfully bagged the baby hyrax, so they could come to their companion's rescue; they dragged Jacob away and helped their fellow hunter to remove the bag from his foot. Luckily the hyrax had released her hold on his foot when she was crammed into the bag, and had obviously become too frightened to bite him again, but even so it must have been an unpleasant experience.

Still shaken with gusts of laughter, which I did my best to conceal, I soothed the wounded Beagle and gave Jacob a good talking to, informing him that he would get only half the price of the capture, owing to his stupidity, and the other half would go to the hunter whose foot he had been so anxious to sacrifice. This decision was greeted with nods and grunts of satisfaction from everyone, including, strangely enough, Jacob himself. Most Africans, I have found, have a remarkably well-developed sense of justice, and will agree heartily with a fair verdict even if it is against themselves.

With order thus restored and first aid rendered to the wounded, we went farther up the valley. After smoking out several caves and holes, with no results, we at last cornered and captured, without bloodshed on either side, a large male hyrax. Having thus got four of the animals, I felt I had had more than my fair share of luck, and that it would be a good idea to return home. We made our way out of the valley, along the edge of the mountain, and then down the gentle slopes of rolling golden grass towards Bafut. When we reached more or less level country we stopped for a smoke and a rest, and as we squatted in the warm grass I glanced back towards the mountains, my attention attracted by a low rumble of thunder. Unnoticed by us, a dark and heavy cloud had drifted across the sky, the shape of a great Persian cat, and had sprawled itself along the crest of the mountains. Its shadow changed them from green and gold to a deep and ugly purple, with harsh black stripes where the valleys lay. The cloud seemed to move, shifting and coiling within itself, and appeared to be padding and kneading the mountain crests like a cat on the arm of a gigantic chair. Occasionally a rent would appear in this nebulous shape, and then it would be pierced by an arrow of sunlight which would illuminate an area of the mountain below with a pure golden light, turning the grass to jade-green patches on the purple flanks of the mountains. With amazing rapidity the cloud grew darker and darker, and seemed to swell as though gathering itself for a spring. Then the lightning began falling like jagged silver icicles, and the mountains shuddered with the vibrations of the thunder that followed.

'Masa, we go walka quick,' said one of the Beagles; 'sometime dat storm go reach us.'

We continued on our way as fast as we could, but we were not fast enough, for the cloud spilled over the mountain top and spread over the sky behind us in a slow motion leap. A cold and agitated wind came hurrying ahead, and close on its heels came the rain, in an almost solid silver curtain that drenched us within the first few seconds. The red earth turned dark and slippery, and the hiss of the rain in the grass made conversation almost impossible. By the time we had gained the outskirts of Bafut our teeth were chattering with cold and our sodden garments were sticking icily to us as we moved. We reached the last stretch of road and the rain dwindled to a fine, drifting spray, and then ceased altogether, while a white mist rose from the sodden earth and broke round our legs like the backwash of an enormous wave.

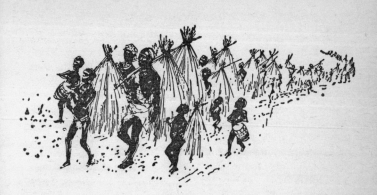

CHAPTER FOUR

The King and the Conga

THE great day of the grass-gathering ceremony arrived at last. Before dawn, when the stars had only just started to fade and dwindle, before even the youngest and most enthusiastic village cockerel had tried his voice, I was awakened by the gentle throb of small drums, laughter and chatter of shrill voices, and the soft scuff of bare feet on the dusty road below the house. I lay and listened to these sounds until the sky outside the window was faintly tinged with the green of the coming day, then I went out on to the veranda to see what was happening.

The mountains that clustered around Bafut were mauve and grey in the dim morning light, striped and patterned with deep purple and black in the valleys, where it was still night. The sky was magnificent, black in the West where the last stars quivered, jade green above me, fading to the palest kingfisher blue at the eastern rim of hills. I leant on the wall of the veranda where a great web of bougainvillaea had grown, like a carelessly flung cloak of brick-red flowers, and looked down the long flight of steps to the road below, and beyond it to the Fon's courtyard. Down the road, from both directions, came a steady stream of people, laughing and talking and beating on small drums when the mood took them. Over their shoulders were long wooden poles, and tied to these with creepers were big conical bundles of dried grass. The children trotted along carrying smaller bundles on thin saplings. They made their way down past the arched opening into the Fon's courtyard and deposited their grass in heaps under the trees by the side of the road. Then they went through the arch into the courtyard, and there they stood about in chattering groups; occasionally a flute and a drum would strike up a brief melody, and then some of the crowd would break into a shuffling dance, amid handclaps and cries of delight from the onlookers. They were a happy, excited, and eager throng.

By the time I had finished breakfast the piles of grass bundles by the roadside were towering skywards, and threatening to overbalance as each new lot was added; the courtyard was now black with people, and they overflowed through the arched door and out into the road. The air was full of noise as the first arrivals greeted the late-comers and chaffed them for their laziness. Children chased each other in and out of the crowd, shrieking with laughter, and hordes of thin and scruffy dogs galloped joyfully at their heels, yelping enthusiastically. I walked down the seventy-five steps to the road to join the crowd, and I was pleased and flattered to find that they did not seem to resent my presence among them, but greeted me with quick, welcoming smiles that swiftly turned to broad grins of delight when I exchanged salutations in pidgin English. I eventually took up a suitable position by the roadside, in the shade of a huge hibiscus bush, scarlet with flowers and filled with the drone of insects. I soon had round me an absorbed circle of youths and children, who watched me silently as I sat and smoked and gazed at the gay crowd that surged past us. Eventually I was run to earth by a panting Ben, who pointed out reproachfully that it was long past lunch-time, and that the delicacy the cook had prepared would undoubtedly be ruined. Reluctantly I left my circle of disciples (who all stood up politely and shook my hand) and followed the grumbling Ben back to the house.

Having eaten, I descended once more to my vantage point

beneath the hibiscus, and continued my anthropological survey of the Bafut people as they streamed steadily past. Apparently during the morning I had been witnessing the arrival of the common or working man. He was, as a rule, dressed in a gaudy sarong twisted tightly round the hips; the women wore the same, though some of the very old ones wore nothing but a dirty scrap of leather at the loins. This, I gathered, was the old style of costume: the bright sarong was a modern idea. Most of the older women smoked pipes – not the short, stubby pipes of the lowland tribes, but ones with long, slender stems, like old-fashioned clay pipes; and they were black with use. This was how the lower orders of Bafut dressed. In the afternoon the council members, the petty chiefs, and other men of substance and importance started to arrive, and there was no mistaking them for just ordinary creatures of the soil. They all wore long, loose-fitting robes of splendid colours, which swished and sparkled as they walked, and on their heads were perched the little flat skull-caps I had noticed before, each embroidered with an intricate and colourful design. Some of them carried long, slender staves of a dark brown wood, covered with a surprisingly delicate tracery of carving. They were all middle-aged or elderly, obviously very conscious of their high office, and each greeted me with great solemnity, shaking me by the hand and saying 'Welcome' several times very earnestly. There were many of these aristocrats and they added a wonderful touch of colour to the proceedings. When I went back to the house for tea I paused at the top of the steps and looked down at the great courtyard: it was a solid block of humanity, packed so tightly together that the red earth was invisible, except in places where some happy dancers cleared a small circle by their antics. Dotted among the crowd I could see the colourful robes of the elders like flowers scattered across a bed of black earth.

Towards evening I was in the midst of the thickest part of the throng, endeavouring to take photographs before the light got too bad, when a resplendent figure made his appearance at my side. His robe glowed with magenta, gold, and green, and in one hand he held a long leather switch. He was the Fon's messenger, he informed me, and, if I was quite ready, he would take me to the Fon for the grass ceremony. Hastily cramming another film into the camera, I followed him through the crowd, watching with admiration as he cut a way through the thickest part by the simple but effective method of slicing with his switch across the bare buttocks that presented themselves so plentifully on all sides. To my surprise the crowd did not seem to take exception to this treatment but yelped and screamed in mock fear, and pushed and stumbled out of our way, all laughing with delight. The messenger led me across the great courtyard, through the arched doorway, along a narrow passage, and then through another arched doorway that brought us out into a honeycomb of tiny courtyards and passages. It was as complicated as a maze, but the messenger knew his way about, and ducked and twisted along passages, through courtyards, and up and down small flights of steps until at length we went through a crumbling brick archway and came out into an oblong courtyard about a quarter of an acre in extent, surrounded by a high red brick wall. At one end of this courtyard grew a large mango tree, and around its smooth trunk had been built a circular raised dais; on this was a big heavily carved chair, and in it sat the Fon of Bafut.

His clothing was so gloriously bright that, for the moment, I did not recognize him. His robe was a beautiful shade of sky blue, with a wonderful design embroidered on it in red, yellow, and white. On his head was a conical red felt hat, to which had been stitched vast numbers of hairs from elephants' tails. From a distance it made him look as though he were wearing a cone-shaped haystack on his head. In one hand he held a fly-whisk, the handle of delicately carved wood and the switch made from the long, black-and-white tail of a colobus monkey – a thick silky plume of hair. The whole very impressive effect was somewhat marred by the Fon's feet: they were resting on a huge elephant tusk – freckled yellow and black with age – that lay before him, and they were clad in a pair of very pointed piebald shoes, topped off by jade-green socks.

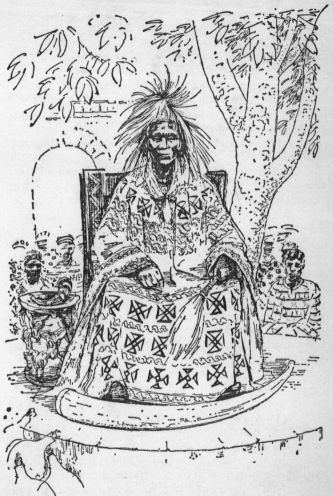

After he had shaken me by the hand and asked earnestly
after my health, a chair was brought for me and I sat down
beside him. The courtyard was lined with various councillors,
petty chiefs, and their half-naked wives, all of them squatting

along the walls on their haunches, drinking out of carved cow-horn flasks. The men's multi-coloured robes made a wonderful tapestry along the red stone wall. To the left of the Fon's throne was a great pile of black calabashes, their necks stuffed with bunches of green leaves, containing mimbo or palm wine, the most common drink in the Cameroons. One of the Fon's wives brought a glass for me, and then lifted a calabash, removed the plug of leaves, and poured a drop of mimbo into the Fon's extended hand. He rolled the liquid round his mouth thoughtfully, and then spat it out and shook his head. Another flask was broached with the same result, and then two more. At last a calabash was found that contained mimbo the Fon considered fine enough to share with me, and the girl filled my glass. Mimbo looks like well-watered milk, and has a mild, faintly sour, lemonade taste which is most deceptive. A really good mimbo tastes innocuous, and thus lures you on to drink more and more, until suddenly you discover that it is not so harmless as you had thought. I tasted my glass of wine, smacked my lips, and complimented the Fon on the vintage. I noticed that all the councillors and petty chiefs were drinking out of flasks made from cow's horn, whereas the Fon imbibed his mimbo from a beautifully carved and polished buffalo horn. We sat there until it was almost dark, talking and gradually emptying the calabashes of mimbo.

Eventually the Fon decided that the great moment for feeding the masses had arrived. We rose and walked down the courtyard between the double ranks of bowing subjects, the men clapping their hands rhythmically, while the women held their hands over their mouths, patting their lips and hooting, producing a noise that I, in my ignorance, had thought to be the prerogative of the Red Indian. We made our way through the doors, passages, and tiny courtyards, the concourse filing behind, still clapping and hooting. As we came out of the archway into the main courtyard there arose from the multitude a deafening roar of approval, accompanied by clapping and drumming. Amid this tumultuous reception the Fon and I walked along the wall to where the Fon's throne had been placed on a leopard skin. We took our seats, the Fon waved his hand, and the feast began.

Through the archway came an apparently endless stream of young men, naked except for small loin-cloths, carrying on their shining and muscular shoulders the various foods for the people. There were calabashes of palm wine and corn beer, huge bunches of plantain and bananas, both green and golden yellow; there was meat in the shape of giant Cane Rats, mongooses, bats and antelope, monkeys and great hunks of python, all carefully smoked and spitted on bamboo poles. Then there were dried fish, dried shrimp and fresh crabs, scarlet and green peppers, mangoes, oranges, pawpaws, pineapples, coconuts, cassava, and sweet potatoes. While this enormous quantity of food was being distributed, the Fon greeted all the headmen, councillors, and chiefs. They would each approach him, then bend double before him and clap their hands three times. The Fon would give a brief and regal nod, and the man would retire backwards. If anyone wanted to address the Fon they had to do so through their cupped hands.

I had by now absorbed quite a quantity of mimbo and was feeling more than ordinarily benign; it seemed to have much the same effect on the Fon. He barked a sudden order, and, to my horror, a table was produced on which reposed two glasses and a bottle of gin, a French brand that I had never heard of, and whose acquaintance I am not eager to renew. The Fon poured out about three inches of gin into a glass and handed it to me; I smiled and tried to look as though gin, neat and in large quantities, was just what I had been wanting. I smelt it gingerly, and found that it was not unlike one of the finer brands of paraffin. Deciding that I really could not face such a large amount undiluted, I asked for some water. The Fon barked out another order, and one of his wives came running, clutching a bottle of Angostura bitters in her hand.

'Beeters!' said the Fon proudly, shaking about two teaspoonfuls into my gin; 'you like gin wit beeters?'

'Yes,' I said with a sickly smile, 'I love gin with bitters.'

The first sip of the liquid nearly burnt my throat out: it was quite the most filthy raw spirits I have ever tasted. Even the Fon, who did not appear to worry unduly about such things, blinked a bit after his first gulp. He coughed vigorously and turned to me, wiping his streaming eyes.

'Very strong,' he pointed out.

Presently, when all the food had been brought out and arranged in huge piles in front of us, the Fon called for silence and made a short speech to the assembled Bafutians, telling them who I was, why I was there, and what I wanted. He ended by explaining to them that they had to procure plenty of animals for me. The crowd listened to the speech in complete silence, and when it had ended a chorus of loud 'Arhhh's!' broke loose, and much hand-clapping. The Fon sat down looking rather pleased with himself, and, carried away by his enthusiasm, he took a long swig at his gin. The result was an anxious five minutes for us all as he coughed and writhed on his throne, tears streaming down his face. He recovered eventually and sat there glaring at the gin in his glass with red and angry eyes. He took another very small sip of it, and rolled it round his mouth, musing. Then he leant over to confide in me.

'Dis gin strong too much,' he said in a hoarse whisper; 'we go give dis strong drink to all dis small-small men, den we go for my house and we drink, eh?'

I agreed that the idea of distributing the gin among the petty chiefs and councillors – the small-small men as the Fon called them – was an excellent one.

The Fon looked cautiously around to make sure we were not overheard; as there were only some five thousand people wedged around us he felt that he could tell me a secret in complete safety. He leant over and lowered his voice to a whisper once more.

'Soon we go for my house,' he said, gleefully; 'we go drink White Horshe.'

He sat back to watch the effect of his words on me. I rolled my eyes and tried to appear overcome with joy at the thought of this treat, while wondering what effect whisky would have on top of mimbo and gin. The Fon, however, seemed satisfied, and presently he called over the small-small men, one by one, and poured the remains of the gin into their cow-horn drinking cups, which were already half filled with mimbo. Never have I given up a drink so gladly. I wondered at the cast-iron stomachs that could face with equanimity, and even pleasure, a cocktail composed of that gin and mimbo. I felt quite sick at the mere thought of it.

Having distributed this rather doubtful largesse among his following, the Fon rose to his feet, amid handclaps, drum-beats, and Red Indian hootings, and led the way back through the intricate web of passages and courts, until we came to his own small villa, almost hidden among his wives' many grass huts, like a matchbox in an apiary. We went inside, and I found myself in a large, low room furnished with easy-chairs and a big table, the wooden floor covered with fine leopard skins and highly coloured, locally made grass mats. The Fon, having done his duty to his people, relaxed in a long chair, and the White Horse was produced; my host smacked his lips as the virginal bottle was uncorked, and gave me to understand that, now the boring duties of state were over, we could start to drink in earnest. For the next two hours we drank steadily, and discussed at great length and in the most complicated detail such fascinating topics as the best type of gun to use on an elephant, what White Horse was made of, why I didn't attend dinners at Buckingham Palace, the Russian question, and so on. After this neither the Fon's questions nor my answers had the skill and delicate construction that we would have liked, so the Fon called for his band, being under the misguided impression that the ravages of strong drink could be dissipated by sweet music. The band came into the court-yard outside and played and danced for a long time, while the Fon insisted that another bottle of White Horse be broached to celebrate the arrival of the musicians. Presently the band formed a half-circle, and a woman did a swaying, shuffling dance and sang a song in a shrill and doleful voice. I could not understand the words, but the song was strangely mournful, and both the Fon and I were deeply affected by it. Eventually the Fon, wiping his eyes, sharply informed the band that they nad better play something else. They had a long discussion among themselves and finally broke into a tune which was the most perfect Conga rhythm imaginable. It was so bright and gay that it quickly revived our spirits, and very soon I was tapping the rhythm out with my foot, while the Fon conducted the band with a glass of White Horse clutched in one hand. Flushed with the Fon's hospitality, and carried away by the tune, an idea came to me.

'The other night you done show me native dance, no be so?' I asked the Fon.

'Na so,' he agreed, stifling a hiccup.

'All right. Tonight you like I go teach you European dance?'

'Ah! my friend,' said the Fon, beaming and embracing me; 'yes, yes, foine, you go teach me. Come, we go for dancing house.'

We rose unsteadily to our feet and made our way to the dance-hall. When we reached it, however, I found that the effort of walking fifty yards had told on my companion; he sank on to his ornate throne with a gasp.

'You go teach all dis small-small men first,' he said, gesturing wildly at the throng of chiefs and councillors, 'den I go dance.'

I surveyed the shuffling, embarrassed crowd of council members that I was supposed to teach, and decided that the more intricate parts of the Conga – which was the jig I proposed to tutor them in – would be beyond them. Indeed, I was beginning to feel that they might even be beyond me. So I decided that I would content myself with showing them the latter part of the dance only, the part where everyone joins into a line and does a sort of follow-my-leader around the place. The whole dance-hall was hushed as I beckoned the two-and-twenty council members to join me on the floor, and in the silence you could hear their robes swishing as they walked. I made them tag on behind me, each holding on to his predecessor's waist; then I gave a nod to the band, who, with great gusto, threw themselves into the conga rhythm, and we were off. I had carefully instructed the pupils to follow my every movement, and this they did. I soon discovered, however, that everything I knew about the Conga had been swamped by the Fon cellars: all I could remember was that somewhere, some time, one gave a kick. So off we went, with the band playing frenziedly, round and round the dance-hall: one, two, three, kick; one, two, three, kick. My pupils had no difficulty in following this simple movement, and we went round the floor in great style, all their robes swishing in unison. I was counting the beats and shouting 'Kick' at the appropriate moment, in order to make the thing simpler for them to follow; apparently they took this to be part of the dance, a sort of religious chant that went with it, for they all started shouting in unison. The effect on our very considerable audience was terrific: screeching with delight, various other members of the Fon's retinue, about forty of his wives, and several of his older offspring, all rushed to join on to the column of dancing councillors, and as each new dancer joined on to the tail he or she also joined the chant.

'One, two three, keek!' yelled the councillors.

'One, two, three, YARR!' yelled the wives.

'On, doo, ree, YARR!' screeched the children.

The Fon was not going to be left out of this dance. He struggled up from his throne and, supported by a man on each side, he tagged on behind; his kicks did not altogether coincide with the rhythmic movement of the rest of us, but he enjoyed himself none the less. I led them round and round the dance-hall until I grew giddy and the whole structure seemed to vibrate with the kicks and yells. Then, feeling that a little fresh air was indicated, I led them out of the door and into the open. Off we went in a tremendous, swaying line, up and down steps, in and out of courtyards, through strange huts – in fact everywhere that offered a free passage. The band, not to be outdone, followed us as we danced, running behind, sweating profusely, but never for one moment losing the tune. At last, more by luck than a sense of direction, I led my followers back into the dance-hall, where we collapsed in a panting, laughing heap. The Fon, who had fallen down two or three

times during our
tour, was escorted back to
his chair, beaming and gasping.
'Na foine dance, dis,' he proclaimed;
'foine, foine!'

'You like?' I asked, gulping for air.

'I like too much,' said the Fon firmly;
'you get plenty power; I never see European dance like dis.'

I was not surprised; few Europeans
in West Africa spend their spare time
teaching the Conga to native chieftains and their courts. I have

no doubt that, if they could have seen me doing that dance,
they would have informed me that I had done more damage
to the White Man's prestige in half an hour than anyone else
had done in the whole history of the West Coast. However,
my Conga appeared to have increased my prestige with the

Fon and his court. 'One, two, three, keek!' murmured the Fon reminiscently; 'na fine song dis.'

'Na very special song,' said I.

'Na so?' said the Fon, nodding his head; 'na foine one.'

He sat on his throne and brooded for a while; the band struck up again and the dancers took the floor; I regained my breath and was beginning to feel rather proud of myself, when my companion woke up suddenly and gave an order. A young girl of about fifteen left the dancers and approached the dais where we sat. She was plump and shining with oil, and clad in a minute loin-cloth which left few of her charms to the imagination. She sidled up to us, smiling shyly, and the Fon leant forward and seized her by the wrist. With a quick pull and a twist he catapulted her into my lap, where she sat convulsed with giggles.

'Na for you, dis woman,' said the Fon, with a lordly wave of one enormous hand, 'na fine one. Na my daughter. You go marry her.'

To say that I was startled means nothing; I was horror-stricken. My host was by now in that happy state that precedes belligerency, and I knew that my refusal would have to be most tactfully put so that I should not undo the good work of the evening. I glanced around helplessly and noticed for the first time what a very large number of the crowd had spears with them. By now the band had stopped playing, and everyone was watching me expectantly. My host was regarding me glassy-eyed. I had no means of telling whether he was really offering me the girl as a wife, or whether this term was used as an euphemism for a more indelicate suggestion. Whichever it was, I had to refuse: quite apart from anything else, the girl was not my type. I licked my lips, cleared my throat, and did the best I could. First, I thanked the Fon graciously for the kind offer of his well-oiled daughter, whose eleven odd stone were at that moment making my knees ache. However, I knew that he was well versed in the stupid customs of my countrymen, and that being so, he knew it was impossible (however desirable) for a man in England to have more than one wife. The Fon nodded wisely at this. Therefore, I went on, I would be forced to refuse his extremely generous offer, for I already had one wife in England, and it would be unlawful, as well as unsafe, to take a second one back with me. If I had not already been married, I went on fluently, there would have been nothing I could have liked better than to accept his gift, marry the girl, and settle down in Bafut for the rest of my life.

To my great relief a loud round of applause greeted my speech, and the Fon wept a bit that this lovely dream could never be realized. During the uproar I eased my dusky girl friend off my lap, gave her a slap on the rump and sent her giggling back to the dance-floor. Feeling that I had undergone quite enough for one night in the cause of diplomatic relations, I suggested that the party break up. The Fon and his retinue accompanied me to the great courtyard and here he insisted on clasping me round the waist and doing the Durrell Conga once more. The crowd fell in behind and we danced across the square, kicking and yelling, frightening the Fruit Bats out of the mango trees, and setting all the dogs barking for miles around. At the bottom of the steps the Fon and I bade each other a maudlin farewell, and I watched them doing an erratic Conga back across the courtyard. Then I climbed up the seventy-five steps, thinking longingly of bed. I was met at the top by a disapproving Ben with a hurricane lamp.

'Sah, some hunter-man done come,' he said.

'What, at this hour?' I asked, surprised, for it was after three.

'Yes, sah. You want I tell um to go?'

'They done bring beef?' I asked hopefully, with visions of some rare specimen.

'No, sah. They want palaver with Masa.'

'All right. Bring um,' I said, sinking into a chair.

Presently Ben ushered in five embarrassed young hunters, all clutching spears. They bowed and said good evening politely. Apparently they had been at the feast that night, and had heard the Fon's speech; as they lived at a village some distance away, they thought they had better see me before they returned home, in order to find out exactly what kind of animals I wanted. I commended their zeal, distributed cigarettes, and brought out books and photographs. We pored over them for a long time, while I told them which creatures I particularly wanted and how much I was willing to pay. Just as they were about to go one young man noticed a drawing lying on my bed that I had not shown them.

'Masa want dis kind of beef?' he asked, pointing.

I peered at the drawing, and then looked at the young man: he seemed to be quite serious about it.

'Yes,' I said emphatically, 'I want dis kind of beef *too much*. Why, you savvay dis beef?'

'Yes, sah, I savvay um,' said the hunter.

I held out the picture to the men.

'Look um fine,' I said.

They all stared at the bit of paper.

'Now, for true, you savvay dis beef?' I asked again, trying to stifle my excitement.

'Yes, sah,' they said, 'we savvay um fine.'

I sat and gazed at them as though they had been beings from another world. Their casual identification of the picture, coming so unexpectedly, had quite startled me, for the drawing depicted a creature that I had long wanted to get hold of, perhaps the most remarkable amphibian in the world, known to scientists as *Trichobatrachus robustus*, and to anyone else as the Hairy Frog.

A word of explanation is called for at this point. On a previous visit to the Cameroons I had set my heart on capturing some of these weird creatures, but without success. I had been operating then in the lowland forests, and all the hunters there to whom I had shown the picture stoutly denied that any such beast existed. They had looked at me pityingly when I insisted, taking it as just another example of the curiously unbalanced outlook of the white man, for did not everyone know that no frog had hair? Animals had hairs, birds had feathers, but frogs had skin and nothing more. Since it was patently obvious to them that the creature did not exist, they did not bother to search for it, in spite of the huge rewards I offered for its capture. What was the use of looking for a mythical monster, a frog with hairs? I had spent many exhausting nights in the forest, wading up and down streams in search of the elusive amphibian, but with no result, and I had come to believe that, in spite of the textbooks, the hunters were right: the creature was not to be found in the lowland forests. I had been so disillusioned by the scorn and derision which any mention of the Hairy Frog had provoked among the lowland tribes, that on my second trip I had omitted to show the drawing, feeling that the highland hunters would be of the same opinion as their relatives in the great forests. Hence my excitement and astonishment when the young hunter, unprompted, had identified the fabulous beast, and moreover wanted to know if I would like some.

I questioned the hunters closely, quivering like an expectant bloodhound. Yes, for the third time, they did know the beast; yes, it did have hair; yes, it was easy to catch. When I asked where it was found they made sweeping gestures, indicating that the woods were full of them. With glittering eyes I asked if they knew of any particular spot where the frogs were to be found. Yes, they knew of a 'small water' some two miles away where there were generally a few to be seen at night. That was enough for me. I rushed out on to the veranda and uttered a roar. The staff came tumbling out of their hut, bleary-eyed, half asleep, and assembled on the veranda.

'Dis hunter man savvay which side I go find dis frog 'e get beer-beer for 'e l'arse,' I explained, 'so we go catch um one time.'

'*Now*, sah?' asked Ben, horrified.

'Yes, now, now, all you go get bag and torch. Quickly, quickly.'

'For night-time?' asked Ben faintly, for he loved his bed.

'Yes, NOW. Don't just stand there yawning, *go and get torches and bags*.'

The staff, reluctant, puffy-eyed, and yawning, shuffled off to obey. Jacob, the cook, stopped for a moment to explain to me that he was a cook and not a hunter, and that he did not see why he should be expected to change his vocation at four o'clock in the morning.

'My friend,' I said firmly, 'if you no get bag and torch in five minutes, tomorrow you no be hunter man *or* cook, savvay?'

Hastily he followed the rest of the staff in search of his frog-hunting equipment. Within half an hour my sleepy band was assembled, and we set off down the dewy road on the hunt for the Hairy Frogs.

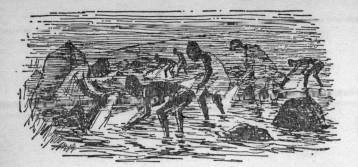

CHAPTER FIVE

Hunt for the Hairy Frogs

IN the dim starlight we made our way down the dusty road, the grass on either side glistening and heavy with dew. There was no moon, which was most fortunate: when you are hunting at night by torchlight a moon is a hindrance and not a help, for it casts strange shadows in which your quarry can disappear, and it enfeebles your torch beam.

The little group of hunters walked ahead, wide awake and eager, while my well-paid staff trailed behind, dragging their toes in the dust and yawning prodigiously. Only Jacob, having decided that, as the hunt was inevitable, he had better make the best of it, walked beside me. Occasionally he would glance over his shoulder with a snort of derision, as a more than usually powerful yawn made itself heard from behind.

'Dis people no get power,' he said scornfully.

'I tink sometime dey done forget I go pay five shillings for dis frog we go hunt,' I explained loudly and clearly. My voice carried well in the still night air, and immediately the yawning and the dragging footsteps ceased as the rear column became very much awake. Five shillings was a large sum to pay for a frog.

'I no forget,' said Jacob, slyly grinning up at me.

'That I do not doubt,' I said severely; 'you're a thoroughly unprincipled West African Shylock.'

'Yes, sah,' Jacob agreed unemotionally. It was impossible

80

to crush him: if he did not understand you he simply played safe and agreed with all you said.

We walked down the road for perhaps a mile and a half, then the hunters turned off on to a narrow path through the long grass, a path that was slippery with dew and that led in an erratic series of zig-zags up the side of a hill. All around us in the damp tangle of long grass the tiny frogs and crickets were calling, like a million Lilliputian metronomes; once a large, pale moth rose, spiralling vaguely from the side of the path, and as it fluttered upwards a nightjar came out of the shadows, swiftly and smoothly as an arrow, and I heard the click of its beak as the moth disappeared. The bird turned and skimmed off down the hillside as silently as it had come. When we reached the crest of the hill the hunters informed me that the small stream they had referred to lay in the valley ahead of us. It was a deep, narrow, shadow-filled cleft that ran between the two smooth, buttock-shaped hills, and the curving line of the stream was marked by a dark fringe of small trees and bushes. As we descended into the gloom of the valley the sound of water came to us, gurgling and clopping among the boulders of its bed, and the surface of the path turned to glutinous clay that made unpleasant sucking noises round our feet as we picked our way down, slipping and sliding.

The stream fled down the valley, slithering down a series of wide, shallow, boulder-strewn steps; at the edge of each step was a diminutive waterfall, perhaps eight feet high, and here the stream gathered itself into a polished column of water and plunged down into a circular pool gouged out among the rocks, where it swirled round and round in a nest of silver bubbles before diving on among the litter of rocks towards the next fall. The long grass curved over the edge of the stream in an uncombed mane of golden hair, and among the glistening boulders grew delicate ferns and tiny plants embedded in thick moss that spread everywhere like a layer of green velvet. On the bank, walking delicately on tip-toe, were numbers of small pink and chocolate crabs, and as our torch beams picked them out they raised their claws menacingly and backed, with infinite caution, down the holes in the red clay that they had dug for themselves. Dozens of minute white moths rose from the long grass as we walked through it, and drifted out across the stream like a cloud of snowflakes. We squatted on the bank to have a smoke and discuss our plan of campaign. The hunters explained that the best place to search for frogs was in the pools at the base of the small waterfalls, but that you also found them under flat rocks in the shallower parts of the stream. I decided that we had better spread out in a line across the stream, and wade up it turning over every movable stone and searching every nook and cranny that might harbour a Hairy Frog. This we did, and for an hour we worked our way steadily uphill towards the source of the stream, splashing through the shallow icy water, slipping on the wet rocks, shining our torches into every hiding-place, and turning over the loose rocks with infinite care.

There were plenty of crabs, scuttling and clicking among the stones, bullet-shaped frogs of bright grass green that leapt into the water with loud plops and startled us; there was a wavering curtain of small moths fluttering everywhere, small bats that flicked in and out of our torch-beams, but no Hairy Frogs. We walked, for the most part, in silence; there were the hundred different voices of the stream as it moved in its bed, the zinging of crickets in the long grass, the occasional cry of a startled bird disturbed by our torch-beams, or the sucking gurgle, followed by a splash, as one of us turned a stone over in deep water. Once when we were negotiating a small cliff over which, like a pulsating lace curtain, hung a waterfall, we were startled by a loud scream and a splash. Directing our battery of lights down to the base of the fall we found that Jacob, who had been last to scale the cliff, had put his foot on a water-snake which lay coiled up in a hollow. In his fright he had attempted to leap in the air, but without much success, for he was clinging precariously to the cliff face some five feet from the ground. He fell into the pool at the base of the falls, and emerged unhurt – but soaking wet and with his teeth chattering from his immersion in the freezing waters.

The eastern skies were turning slowly from black to pale green with the coming of dawn, and still we had not found our elusive amphibian. The hunters, who were acutely depressed by our failure, explained that it was useless continuing the search once it was light, for then the frog would not show itself. This meant that we had some two hours left in which to track down the beast and capture it, and, though we continued on our way up the stream, I was convinced that our luck was out and that we would not be successful. At last, damp, cold, and dispirited, we came to a broad, flat valley filled with great boulders through which the stream picked its way like a snake. At certain points it had formed deep, quiet pools among the rocks, and, as the ground was flat, the movement of the waters was slow and even, and the stream had doubled its width. The boulders were strewn haphazardly about, all tilted at peculiar angles like giant archaic gravestones, black under the starry sky. Each one was tapestried with moss, and hung with the sprawling plants of wild begonias.

We had moved about half-way up this valley when I decided to break off for a cigarette. I came to a small pool that lay like a black mirror ringed round with tall rocks, and choosing a smooth dry stone to sit on I switched off my torch and sat down to enjoy my smoke. The torch-beams of my retinue twinkled and flashed among the rocks as they continued up the valley, and the splashing of their feet in the water was soon lost among the many night sounds around me. When I had finished my cigarette, I flipped the butt into the air so that it swooped like a glowing firefly and fell into the pool, where it extinguished itself with a hiss. Almost immediately afterwards something jumped into the pool with a loud plop, and the smooth black waters were netted with a thousand silver ripples. I switched on my torch quickly and shone it on the surface of the water, but there was nothing to be seen. Then I flashed the beam along the moss-covered rocks which formed the lip of the pool. There, not a yard from where I was sitting, squatting on the extreme edge of a rock, sat a great, gleaming, chocolate-coloured frog, his fat thighs and the sides of his body covered with a tangled pelt of something that looked like hair.

I sat there hardly daring to breathe, for the frog was perched on the extreme edge of the rock, overhanging the pool; he was alert and suspicious, his legs bunched ready to jump. If he was frightened, he would leap straight off the rock and into the dark waters, and then there would be no hope of catching him. For perhaps five minutes I remained as immobile as the rocks around me, and gradually, as he got used to the light, the Hairy Frog relaxed. Once he shifted his position slightly, blinking his moist eyes, and I was filled with panic thinking that he was going to jump. But he settled down again and I sighed with relief. As I sat there I was busy working out a plan: first, I had to switch the torch from my right to my left hand without disturbing him; then I had to lean forward until my hand was near enough to his fat body to risk grabbing at him. Shifting the torch caused me acute anguish, for he watched the manoeuvre with an alert and suspicious eye; when I had achieved the change I sat quietly for a few minutes to allow him to settle down again, then, with great caution, I moved my cupped hand slowly towards him. Inch by inch I moved until my hand was hanging just above him; then I took a deep breath and grabbed. As my hand swooped downwards the frog jumped, but he was not quite quick enough and my grasping fingers caught him by one slippery hind leg. But he was not going to give up his liberty without a fight, and he uttered a loud screaming gurk, and kicked out frantically with his free hind leg, scraping his toes across the back of my hand. As he did so, I felt as though it had been scratched with several needles, and on the skin of the back of my hand appeared several deep grooves which turned red with the welling blood. I was so astonished at this unexpected attack from a creature which I had thought to be completely harmless, that I must have relaxed my hold slightly. The frog gave an extra hard kick and a wriggle, his moist leg slid through my fingers, there was a plop as he hit the water and the ripples danced. My Hairy Frog had escaped.

My heart, if I can so describe it, was too full for words. An extensive collection of lurid descriptive phrases which I had accumulated over the years seemed anaemic and inadequate to describe this catastrophe. I tried one or two, but they were a very weak indication of how I felt. After all this time I had

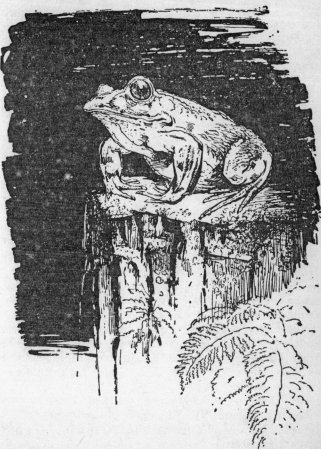

come face to face with a Hairy Frog, after being told that it did not exist; after many hours of fruitless search, I had actually had the beast in my grasp, and then, through my own stupidity, had let it get away. I clambered on to a tall rock to see where my hunters had got to; I could see their lights flashing a quarter of a mile away down the valley, and I uttered the prolonged yodelling call that the hunters use to communicate with each other. When they answered me, I shouted that they were to hurry back, as I had found the beef we were looking for. Then I climbed down and examined the pool carefully. It was perhaps ten feet long and about five feet across at the widest point. It was fed and emptied through two very narrow channels among the rocks, and I decided that if we blocked these, and the frog was still in the pool, we stood a fair chance of recapturing him. When my panting hunters arrived I explained what had happened, and they clicked their fingers and groaned with annoyance upon learning that the frog had escaped. However, we set to work, and soon we had blocked the entrance and exit channels of the pool with piles of flat stones. Then two of the hunters stood on the rocks and shone our battery of torches into the pool so that we could see what we were doing. First, I tested the depth of the water with the long handle of the butterfly net, and found that it was about two feet deep; the bottom of the pool was of coarse gravel and small stones, a terrain that provided ample hiding-places for the frog. Jacob, myself, and two hunters then removed all the garments we had on and slid into the icy water: Jacob and I at one end of the pool, and the two hunters at the other. Slowly we moved down towards each other, bent double, feeling with our fingers and toes in every crack, turning over every stone. Presently, when we had worked to the centre of the pool, one of the hunters gave a yelp of delight and grabbed wildly at something under the water, almost losing his balance and falling on his face.

'Na whatee, na whatee?' we all asked excitedly.

'Na flog,' spluttered the hunter, 'but 'e done run.'

'You no get hand?' inquired Jacob wrathfully through chattering teeth.

''E done run for Masa,' said the hunter, pointing in my direction.

As he spoke, I felt something moving near my bare foot, and I bent down and groped frantically under the water. At the same moment, Jacob uttered a shrill scream and dived under the water, and one of the hunters was frantically grabbing at something between his legs. My hand felt a smooth, fat body burrowing in the gravel near my toes, and I grabbed at it; at the same moment, Jacob reappeared above the water, spitting and gasping and waving one arm triumphantly, his hand clasped firmly round a fat frog. He splashed through the water towards me to show me his capture, and as he reached me I straightened up with my own prize caught in my cupped hands. I glanced hurriedly between my fingers and had a quick glimpse of the frog's thick thighs covered with a mat of the hair-like substance; it was a Hairy Frog. Then I looked at Jacob's capture, and found that he had caught one also. After congratulating each other, we cautiously placed out frogs in a deep, soft cloth bag, and tied up the mouth of it carefully. Just as we had done this, the hunter who had been groping wildly between his legs straightened up with a roar of delight, swinging yet another Hairy Frog by the leg.

Warmed and encouraged by our success, we plunged back into the pool once again and searched it carefully, but we found no more frogs. By now the rim of the eastern horizon was a pale powder blue, flecked with gold, and in the sky above us the remaining stars were flickering and dying as stripes of jade green spread across the sky. It was obviously too late to continue with our hunt, but I was well pleased with the results. As the Africans crouched on the rocks, laughing and chattering, smoking the cigarettes I had distributed, I dried myself, rather inadequately, with my handkerchief and put on my dew-soaked clothes. My head was aching savagely, partly, I think, because of the excitement of the capture, but principally owing to the party I had had with the Fon. However, with the glow of triumph enveloping me I cared not for the cold dampness of my clothes, nor for my aching head. The bag with the Hairy Frogs inside I dipped into the pool until it was sodden and cool, then I wrapped it in wet grass and placed it in the bottom of the basket.

As we reached the top of the hill, the sun rose above the distant mountains and flooded the world with a brittle, golden light. The long grass was bent and heavy with dampness, and a thousand tiny spiders had spun their nets among the stalks, and the nets had dredged up from the night a rich haul of dewdrops

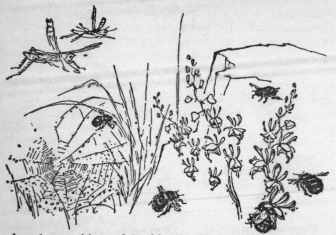

that shone white and ice blue in the sun. Dozens of great locusts leapt up from under our feet and sped over the grass in a whirring glitter of magenta wings; and some fat bumble bees, electric blue and as furry as bears, formed a humming choir over a group of pale yellow orchids growing in the shelter of a large rock. The air was fresh and cool, full of the scent of flowers, grass, earth, and dew. The hunters, happy in the knowledge that the night's activities had been successful, broke into song as they picked their way down the path in single file; a lilting Bafutian melody that they rendered with great verve; the staff joined in, and Jacob beat a gentle tattoo on a collecting tin by way of accompaniment. Thus we marched back to Bafut, singing loudly, Jacob working out more and more complicated rhythms on his improvised drum.

My first job, when we at last reached home, was to prepare a deep tin to house the frogs; this I filled with fresh water, and placed a number of stones at the bottom to act as cover for them. I put two of them into this tin, but the third I placed in a large jam jar. While I had my breakfast, the jam jar rested on the table, and between mouthfuls I contemplated my capture with adoring eyes.

My Hairy Frog was, as frogs go, quite large: with his legs

tucked neatly in he would have fitted on to a saucer without very much room left over. His head was broad and rather flat, with very protuberant eyes and a mouth with an extraordinarily wide gape. The ground colour of the upper parts was a deep chocolate brown, mottled dimly in places with darker brown, almost black markings; the underside was white, flushed with pink on the lower belly and the inside of the thighs. The eyes were very large, jet black netted with a fine filigree of golden marks. The most astonishing thing about the creature – the hair – was confined to the sides of the body and the thighs, where it grew thick and black, about a quarter of an inch long. This adornment is not really hair at all, but consists of fine, elongated filaments of skin, which on close examination resemble the tentacles of a sea anemone. Until you examine the creature closely, however, the illusion that its hind-quarters are clothed in a thick

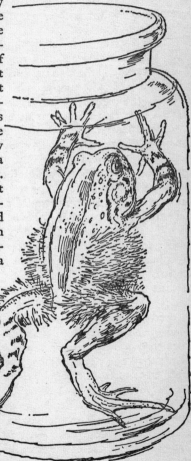

layer of fur is complete. In the water the hair stands out,
floating like weed, and so is seen to the best advantage; when
the frog is out of water the hair takes on a tangled, jelly-like
look.

There has been much controversy, ever since the frog was
first discovered, over the exact use of this curious hirsute decoration, but it is now believed that the filaments act as an aid
to respiration. All frogs breathe, to a certain extent, through
their skins: that is to say, the skin absorbs oxygen from the
moisture on the creature's body. In this way a frog has, so to
speak, two breathing apparatuses – the skin and the lungs.
Thus, by breathing through the skin a frog can stay submerged
in the water for quite considerable periods. In the case of the
Hairy Frog, the great number of filaments give it a much increased skin area, and so must aid its respiration a good deal.
There was considerable doubt originally as to the precise function of the Hairy Frog's hairs, owing to the fact that only the
male is hairy; the female is smooth-skinned like any ordinary
frog. Thus it appeared as though the hairs were purely orna-
mental rather than useful, for it seemed ridiculous to suppose
that the male was so short-winded that he needed hair to enable him to breathe properly, while the female pursued a hair-
less and well-aerated existence. This unusual discrepapcy was,
however, soon explained: it was found that the male spent his
life submerged in water, whereas the female led a purely
terrestrial existence for the greater part of the year, only going
to water during the mating season. So was the mystery explained – the female on land, using her lungs to breathe with
for the most part; whereas her husband in his watery lair
found the hairs a very useful addition, for much of his time
was spent beneath the water.

Next to its hairiness, the most curious thing about this frog
is that it possesses, in the fleshy toes of each hind foot, a set of
long, semi-transparent white claws; these claws, like those of a
cat, are retractile, and when not in use disappear back into the
sheaths in the toes. That these claws are sharp and useful had
been proved to me by the scratches on my hand. I should
imagine that the use of these weapons is twofold: first as a

means of defence, and secondly as a useful tool which enables the amphibian to cling to the slippery rocks in the fast-running streams which it inhabits. Whenever the frogs were picked up they would kick out frantically with their hind legs, and the claws would appear from their sheaths; they would at the same time utter their curious screaming grunts, a cross between the cries of a contented pig and tortured mouse, a sound astonishingly loud and inclined to be very startling when you were not expecting it.

My Hairy Frogs settled down very nicely in their large tin, and, after numerous night hunts, I added to their number until I had seven of them, all males with the most luxuriant backsides. For many weeks I searched high and low to try to find some females to go with them, but without success. Then, one day, a dear old lady who looked about ninety-five appeared on the veranda, carrying two calabashes: in one was a pair of shrews, and in the other was a large female Hairy Frog. This was the only female of the species that I ever obtained, and she was accordingly given special care and attention. She was similar to the males in appearance, except that her skin was drier and slightly rougher, and her colouring was a bright brick-red with chocolate flecks. She settled down quite happily with her seven suitors, and even adopted their habits. During the day they all lay in the water, almost completely submerged, ready to dive to the bottom of the tin should anyone approach; at night, however, they grew braver, and climbed out on to the rocks I had put in there for them, where they would sit gulping at each other with vacant expressions. During all the time I had them in Africa, and on the long voyage back to England, the frogs stubbornly refused to eat any of the tempting delicacies I put before them. But as they were extremely fat, this long fast did not unduly worry me, for most reptiles can go for long periods without food and be none the worse for it.

When the time came for me to leave Bafut and travel down to the base camp, and then on to the coast, I packed the frogs in a shallow wooden box filled with wet banana leaves. The box had to be shallow, for otherwise the frogs when scared would jump wildly into the air and bang their delicate noses on the wooden top; in a shallow box, however, they got no chance of doing this. They caused me considerable trouble on the way down from Bafut, and many anxious moments: in the highlands the climate is cool and pleasant, but as you descend into the forested lowlands it is like entering a Turkish bath, and the frogs did not like this change at all. When I opened the box, during one of our halts on the way down, I was horrified to find all my Hairy Frogs lying in the bottom, limp and apparently lifeless. I rushed frantically down into a nearby ravine and plunged the box into a stream. The cool waters gradually revived four of the frogs, but three were too far gone and soon died. This left me with three males and the female. I had to stop the lorry every two or three miles for the rest of the journey while I ducked the frog box into a stream to revive its inmates; and it was only in this fashion that I managed to get them to base camp alive. On arrival, however, I discovered another problem: the Hairy Frogs had not been able to jump and damage their noses, but they had tried to burrow into the corners of the box, and had thus managed to rub all the skin off their noses and upper lips. This was most serious, for once the delicate skin on a frog's nose is damaged it very soon develops a nasty sore on the spot, which spreads like a rodent ulcer, and can eventually eat away the whole nose and lip. Hastily, I had to create a new box for the frogs to live in; this one was also shallow, but it was completely padded inside, top, bottom, and sides, with soft cloth stuffed with cotton wool. The box resembled a small padded cell. In this the Hairy Frogs did very well, since, whether they jumped or burrowed, they could not injure themselves on the soft surface. By keeping them drier than usual I managed to heal up their scraped noses, but they always had faint white scars on the skin afterwards.

When we finally left the base camp and travelled down to the coast to catch the ship, the journey was a nightmare. It was incredibly hot, and the Hairy Frogs' box dried up very rapidly. I tried keeping it in a tin full of water, but the roads were so bad that most of the water sloshed out inside the first half mile. The only alternative to this was to stop the lorry at a stream every half-hour or so and give the box a thorough soaking.

Yet in spite of this one of the males succumbed, so that only three Hairy Frogs arrived on board ship. The cool sea-breeze soon revived them, and they seemed fit enough, though very thin, owing to their self-imposed fast. The fast continued until they reached England, and for some time after they were installed in the Reptile House at London Zoo. This Curator, as I had done, tried to tempt them with all sorts of delicious tit-bits, but they still refused to eat. Then one day, more or less as a last resort, he put some pink newly born white mice into the cage with them, and to his surprise the frogs fell on them and devoured the lot as though baby mice were their favourite food. From then onwards they lived entirely on this mammalian diet, refusing all the usual froggy foods like locusts and mealworms. It seems highly improbable that they live exclusively on baby mice in the wild state, so it must be that the mice resembled the food that they were used to eating, though what that might be remains shrouded in mystery.

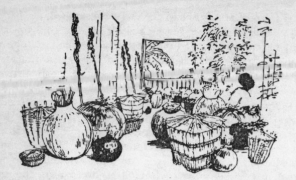

CHAPTER SIX

Snakes and Shillings

THE Fon's speech at the grass-gathering ceremony produced the most astonishing and immediate results. The next afternoon I was endeavouring to dissipate the effects of the Fon's party, and the subsequent frog hunt, by lying down for a couple of hours and catching up on some sleep. When I awoke, I decided that some tea would help to restore me to a more amiable frame of mind, so I staggered off the bed and made my way to the door, intending to shout my instructions down to the kitchen from the veranda. I opened the door and then stopped dead, wondering if I was dreaming, for the whole veranda was literally covered with a weird assortment of sacks, palm-leaf baskets, and calabashes, all of which shook and quivered gently, while leaning up against the wall were four or five long bamboos to the ends of which were tied writhing and infuriated snakes. The veranda looked more like a native market than anything else. At the top of the steps squatted Jacob, scowling at me disapprovingly.

'Masa wake up?' he said mournfully, 'why Masa wake up?'

'What's all this?' I asked, waving my hand at the collection of bags and baskets.

'Beef,' said Jacob succinctly.

I examined the snakes' bonds to make sure they were secure. 'Which man done bring dis beef?' I asked, feeling rather stunned by the profusion of arrivals.

'Dis men done bring um,' said Jacob laconically, gesturing down the steps behind him. I stepped over to where he sat and saw that the seventy-five steps up to the villa, and a good deal of the road beyond, was jammed with a great variety of Bafutians of all ages and both sexes. There must have been about a hundred and fifty of them, and they gazed up at me, unmoving and strangely quiet. As a rule a small group of four or five Africans can make more noise than any other race on earth, yet this great crowd might have been composed of deaf mutes for all the sound it was making. The silence was uncanny.

'What's the matter with them?' I asked Jacob.

'Sah?'

'Why dey no make noise, eh?'

'Ah!' said Jacob, light dawning, 'I done tell um Masa 'e sleep.'

This was the first of many examples I was to have of the courtesy and good manners of the Bafut people. For nearly two hours, I discovered, they had sat there in the hot sun, curbing their natural exuberance so that my slumbers might not be disturbed.

'Why you no wake me before?' I said to Jacob; 'you no savvay na bad ting for dis beef to wait, eh?'

'Yes, sah. Sorry, sah.'

'All right, let's get on with it and see what they've brought.'

I picked up the first basket and peered into it: it contained five mice with pale ginger fur, white tummies, and long tails. I handed the basket to Jacob, who carried it to the top of the steps and held it aloft.

'Who done bring dis beef?' he shouted.

'I done bring um,' called an old woman shrilly. She fought her way up on to the veranda, bargained with me breathlessly for five minutes, and then fought her way down the steps again, clutching her money.

The next basket contained two delightful little owls. They were speckled grey and black, and the area round the eyes was pure white with a black rim, so that they looked as though they were wearing large horn-rimmed glasses. They clicked their beaks at me, and lowered their long eyelashes over their fierce golden eyes when they saw me, and as I tried to pick them up they rolled over on to their backs, presenting their large talons,

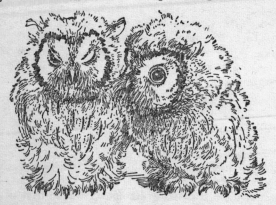

and uttering loud screams. They were quite young, and in places were still clad in the cottonwool-like down of infancy, so that they looked as if they had both been caught in a snow-storm. I can never resist owls at the best of times, but these two babies were quite adorable. They were White-faced Scops Owls, and something quite new to my collection, so I had an excellent reason for buying them.

The next item was a squirrel who created a considerable diversion. He was confined in a palm-leaf bag, and as soon as I opened it he shot out like a jack-in-the-box, bit my hand, and then galloped off across the veranda. Jacob gave chase, and as he drew near, the squirrel suddenly darted to one side and then ran down the steps, weaving his way skilfully through the dozens of black legs that stood there. The panic he created was tremendous: those on the first step leapt into the air as he rushed at their feet, lost their balance, and fell backwards against those on the next step. They, in turn, fell against the ones below them, who went down like grass before a scythe. In a matter of seconds the steps were covered with a tangled

mass of struggling bodies, with arms and legs sticking out at
the oddest angles. I quite thought that the unfortunate squirrel
would be crushed to death under this human avalanche, but to
my surprise he appeared at the bottom of the steps apparently
unhurt, flipped his tail a couple of times and set off down the
road at a brisk trot, leaving behind him a scene which looked
like a negro version of the Odessa steps massacre. At the top
of the steps I was fuming impotently and struggling to push
my way through the tangle of Africans, for the squirrel was a
rarity, and I was determined that he should not escape. Half-
way down someone clutched my ankle and I collapsed abruptly
on top of a large body which, judging from the bits I could see,
was female. I glanced desperately down at the road as I en-
deavoured to regain my feet, and to my joy I saw a band of
some twenty young men approaching. Seeing the squirrel,
they stopped short, whereupon the creature sat up and sniffed
at them suspiciously.

'You!' I roared, 'you dere for de road . . . catch dat beef.'

The young men put down their bundles and advanced determinedly upon the squirrel, who took one look at them and
then turned and fled. They set off in hot pursuit, each resolved
that he should be the one to recapture the rodent. The squirrel
ran well, but he was no match for the long legs of his pursuers.
They drew level with him in a tight bunch, their faces grim and
set. Then, to my horror, they launched themselves at my
precious specimen in a body, and for the second time the
squirrel disappeared under a huge pile of struggling Africans.
This time, I thought, the poor beast really *would* be crushed, but
that squirrel seemed indestructible. When the heap in the road
had sorted itself out a bit, one of the young men stood up holding the chattering and panting squirrel by the scruff of its neck.

'Masa!' he called, beaming up at me, 'I done catch um!'

I threw down a bag for him to put the animal in, and then it
was passed up the steps to me. Hastily I got the beast into a
cage so that I could examine him to make sure he was not
damaged in any way, but he seemed all right except that
he was in an extremely bad temper. He was a Black-eared
Squirrel, perhaps one of the most beautiful of the Cameroon

squirrels. His upper parts were a deep olive green, while his belly was a rich yellow-orange. Along his sides were a series of white spots, set in a line from shoulder to buttocks, and there was a rim of black fur marking the edge of each ear, making him look as though he had never washed behind them. But the most beautiful part of his furry anatomy was his tail. This was long and tremendously bushy: the upper parts were a brindled greeny-brown, while the underparts were the most vivid flame-orange imaginable. Placed in a cage he flipped this dazzling tail at me once or twice, and then squatted down to the stern task of devouring a mango which I had put in there for him. I watched him fondly, thinking what a lucky escape he had had, and how pleased I was to have got him. If I had known what trouble he was going to cause in the future I might have viewed his arrival with considerably less excitement.

I turned my attention back to the various containers that littered the veranda, and picked up a large calabash at random. As usual, its neck was stuffed with a tightly packed plug of green leaves; I removed these and peered into the depths, but the calabash was so capacious and so dark that I could not see what was inside. I carried it to the head of the steps and held it up.

'Which side de man who done bring dis calabash?' I asked.

'Na me, sah, na me!' shouted a man half-way down the steps.

It was always a source of astonishment to me how the Africans could distinguish their own calabashes among hundreds of others. Except for a difference in size I could never tell one from the other, but the Africans knew at a glance which was theirs and which belonged to some other hunter.

'What beef 'e dere-dere for inside?' I asked, negligently swinging the calabash by its cord.

'Snake, sah,' said the man, and I hastily replaced the plug of green leaves.

'What kind of snake, my friend?'

'Na Gera, sah.'

I consulted my list of local names and found this meant a

Green-leaf Viper. These were common and beautiful snakes in Bafut, and I already had quite a number of them. They were about eighteen inches long, a startlingly bright grass green in colour, with canary-yellow bellies and broad diagonal white stripes along their sides. I carried the calabash over to empty the new arrival into the shallow, gauze-topped box in which I kept vipers. Now, emptying a snake from a calabash into a cage is one of the simplest of operations, providing you observe one or two rudimentary rules. First, make sure that any inmates of the cage are far away from the door. This I did. Secondly, make sure how many snakes you have in the calabash before starting to shake them out. This I omitted to do.

I opened the door of the cage, unplugged the mouth of the calabash and began to shake gently. Sometimes it requires quite a lot of shaking to get a snake out of a calabash, for he will coil himself round inside, and press himself against the sides, making it difficult to dislodge him. Jacob stood behind me, breathing heavily down my neck, and behind him stood a solid wall of Africans, watching open-mouthed. I shook the calabash gently, and nothing happened. I shook it a bit harder, with the same result. I had never known a viper cling with such tenacity to the interior of a receptacle. Becoming irritated, I gave the calabash a really vigorous shaking, and it promptly broke in half. An intricately tangled knot of Green-leaf Vipers, composed of about half a dozen large, vigorous, and angry snakes, fell out on to the cage with what can only be described as a sickening thud.

They were plaited together in such a large and solid ball that instead of falling through the door and into the cage, they got jammed half-way, so that I could not slam the door on them. Then, with a fluid grace which I had no time to admire, they disentangled themselves and wriggled determinedly over the edge of the door and on to the floor. Here they spread out fanwise with an almost military precision, and came towards us. Jacob and the Africans who had been jammed behind him disappeared with the startling suddenness of a conjuring trick. I could hardly blame them, for none of them was wearing shoes. But I was not clad to gallivant with a tribe of vipers either, for

99

I was wearing shorts and a pair of sandals. My only armament, moreover, consisted of the two halves of the broken calabash, which is not the most useful thing to have when tackling a snake. Leaving the snakes in sole charge of the veranda, I shot into my bedroom. Here I found a stick, and then went cautiously out on to the veranda again. The snakes had scattered widely, so they were quite easy to corner, pin down with the stick, and then pick up. One by one I dropped them into the cage, and then shut and locked the door with a sigh of relief. The Africans reappeared just as suddenly as they had disappeared, all chattering and laughing and clicking their fingers as they described to each other the great danger they had been in. I fixed the snake-bringer with a very cold eye.

'You!' I said, 'why you no tell me dere be plenty snake for inside dat calabash, eh?'

'Wah!' he said, looking surprised, 'I done tell Masa dere be snake for inside.'

'Snake, yes. *One* snake. You no tell me dere be six for inside.'

'I done tell Masa dere be snake for inside,' he said indignantly.

'I done ask you what beef you done bring,' I explained patiently, 'and you say, "snake". You no say dere be six snake. How you tink I go savvay how many snake you bring, eh? You tink sometime I get juju for my eye and I go savvay how many snake you done catch?'

'Stupid man,' said Jacob, joining in the fray. 'Sometime dis snake bite Masa, and Masa go die. Den how you go do, eh?'

I turned on Jacob.

'I noticed that you were conspicuous by your absence, my noble and heroic creature.'

'Yes, sah!' said Jacob, beaming.

It was not until quite late that evening that the last hunter had been paid, and I was left with such a weird assortment of live creatures on my hands that it took me until three o'clock the following morning to cage them. Even so, there were five large rats left over, and no box from which to make a cage. I was forced to release them in my bedroom, where they spent the entire night trying to gnaw through the leg of the table.

The next morning when I arose and cleaned out and fed my now considerable collection, I thought that probably nothing more would turn up that day. I was wrong. The Bafutians had obviously thrown themselves wholeheartedly into the task of providing me with specimens, and by ten o'clock the road-way and the seventy-five steps were black with people, and in desperation I had to bargain for the creatures. By lunch-time it was obvious that the supply of animals had far exceeded my store of wood and boxes to make cages for them, so I was forced to employ a team of small boys to tour Bafut, buying up any and every box or plank of wood they could find. The prices I had to pay for boxes were exorbitant, for to the African any sort of receptacle, be it a bottle, an old tin or a box, was worth its weight in gold.

By four o'clock that evening both the staff and I were ex-hausted, and we had been bitten so many times and in so many places by such a variety of creatures that any additional bites went almost unnoticed. The whole villa was overflowing with animals, and they squeaked and chirruped, rattled and bumped in their calabashes, baskets, and sacks while we worked furiously to make the cages for them. It was one of those twenty-four hours that one prefers to forget. By midnight we were all so tired we could hardly keep awake, and there were still some ten cages to be made; a large pot of tea, heavily laced with whisky, gave us a sort of spurious enthusiasm for our task that carried us on, and at two-thirty the last nail was driven in and the last animal released into its new quarters. As I crawled into bed, I was horribly aware of the fact that I should have to be up at six the next morning if I wanted to have everything cleaned and fed by the time the next influx of specimens began.

The next day was, if anything, slightly worse than the pre-ceding one, for the Bafutians started to arrive before I had fin-ished attending to the collection. There is nothing quite so nerve-racking as struggling to clean and feed several dozen creatures when twenty or thirty more have arrived in airless and insanitary containers and are crying out for attention. As I watched out of the corner of my eye the pile of calabashes and baskets growing on the veranda, so the number of cages that I had still to clean and attend to seemed to multiply, until I felt rather as Hercules must have felt when he got his first glimpse of the Augean stables.

When I had finished the work, before buying any fresh specimens I made a speech to the assembled Bafutians from the top of the steps. I pointed out that in the last couple of days they had brought me a vast quantity of beef of all shapes, sizes, and descriptions. This proved that the Bafutians were by far the best hunters I had come across, and I was very grateful to them. However, I went on, as they would realize, there was a limit to the amount of beef I could purchase and house in any one day. So I would be glad if they would desist from hunting for the space of three days, in order that my caging and food supply might catch up with them. There was no sense, I pointed out, in my buying beef from them if it was going to die for lack of adequate housing; that was just simply a waste of money. The African is nothing if not a business man, and at this remark the nodding of heads sent a ripple over the crowd, and a chorus of 'Arrrrr!' arose. Having thus driven the point home, and, I hoped, given myself three days' respite, I purchased the animals they had brought and once more set about the task of cage-building.

At four o'clock the caging was under control, and I was having a break for a cup of tea. As I leant on the veranda rail I saw the arched doorway in the red brick wall fly open and the Fon appeared. He strode across the great courtyard with enormous strides, his robes fluttering and hissing as he moved. He was scowling worriedly and muttering to himself. As it was obvious that he was on his way to pay me a visit, I went down the steps to meet him.

'Iseeya, my friend,' I said politely as he reached me.

'My friend!' he said, enveloping my hand in his and peering earnestly into my face, 'some man done tell me you no go buy beef again. Na so?'

'No be so,' I said.

'Ah! Good, good!' he said in a relieved voice. 'Sometime I fear you done get enough beef an' you go lef' dis place.'

'No, no be so,' I explained. 'People for Bafut savvay hunting too much, and dey done bring me so many beef I no get box for put um. So I done tell all dis people dey no go hunt for three days, so I get chance for make box for put all dis beef.'

'Ah! I savvay,' said the Fon, smiling at me affectionately. 'I tink sometime you go lef' us.'

'No, I no go lef' Bafut.'

The Fon peered anxiously round in a conspiratorial fashion, and then, draping one arm lovingly round my shoulders, he drew me down the road.

'Ma friend,' he said in a hoarse whisper, 'I done find beef for you. Na fine beef, na beef you never get.'

'What kind of beef?' I asked curiously.

'Beef,' said the Fon explicitly, 'you go like *too much*. We go catch um now, eh?'

'You never catch um yet?'

'No, my friend, but I savvay which side dey de hide.'

'All right. We go look um now, eh?'

'Yes, yes, foine!' said the Fon.

Eagerly he led me across the great courtyard, through a maze of narrow passages, until we reached a small hut.

'Wait here small time, my friend, I go come,' he said, and then disappeared hurriedly into the gloom of the hut. I waited outside, wondering where he had gone to and what kind of beef it was that he had discovered. He had an air of mystery about him which made the whole thing rather intriguing.

When he eventually reappeared, for a moment I did not recognize him. He had removed his robes, his skull-cap, and his sandals, and was now naked except for a small and spotlessly white loin-cloth. In one hand he held a long and slender spear. His thin, muscular body gleamed with oil, and his feet were bare. He approached me, twirling his spear professionally, beaming with delight at my obvious surprise.

'You done get new hunter man,' he said, chuckling; 'now you fit call me Bafut Beagle, no be so?'

'I tink dis hunter man be best for all,' I said, grinning at him.

'I savvay hunting fine,' he said, nodding. 'Sometime my people tink I get ole too much for go bush. My friend, if some man get hunting for 'e eye, for 'e nose, an' for 'e blood, 'e *never* get ole too much for go bush, no be so?'

'You speak true, my friend,' I said.

He led me out of the environs of his compound, along the road for perhaps half a mile, and then branched off through some maize-fields. He walked at a great pace, twirling his spear and humming to himself, occasionally turning to grin at me with mischievous delight illuminating his features. Presently we left the fields, passed through a small thicket of mimbo palms, dark and mysterious and full of the rustling of the fronds, and then started to climb up the golden hillside. When we reached the top, the Fon paused, stuck his spear into the ground, folded his arms, and surveyed the view. I had stopped a little way down the hillside to collect some delicately coloured snails; when I had arrived at the top, the Fon appeared to have gone into a trance. Presently he sighed deeply, and, turning towards me, smiled and swept his arms wide.

'Na my country dis,' he said, 'na foine, dis country.'

I nodded in agreement, and we stood there in silence for a few minutes and looked at the view. Below us lay a mosaic of small fields, green and silver and fawn, broken up by mimbo palm thickets and an occasional patch of rust red where the earth of a field had been newly hoed. This small area of cultivation was like a coloured handkerchief laid on the earth and forgotten, surrounded on all sides by the great ocean of mountains, their crests gilded and their valleys smudged with shadow by the falling sun. The Fon gazed slowly round, an expression on his face that was a mixture of affection and child-like pleasure. He sighed again, a sigh of satisfaction.

'Foine!' he murmured. Then he plucked his spear from the earth and led the way down into the next valley, humming tunefully to himself.

The valley was shallow and flat, thickly overgrown with a wood of small stunted trees, some only about ten feet high.

Many of them were completely invisible under immense cloaks of convolvulus, squat towers of trembling leaves and ivory-coloured flowers. The valley had captured the sunshine of the day, and the warm air was heavy and sweet with the scent of flowers and leaves. A sleepy throbbing drone came from a thousand bees that hovered round the flowers; a tiny anonymous bird let a melodious trickle of song fill the valley, and then stopped suddenly, so that the only sound was the blurred singing of the bees again, as they hovered round the trees or waddled up the smooth tunnel of the convolvulus flowers. The Fon surveyed the trees for a moment, and then moved quietly through the grass to a better vantage point, where our view into the wood was not so clogged with convolvulus.

'Na for here we go see beef,' he whispered, pointing at the trees; 'we sit down an' wait small time.'

He squatted down on his haunches and waited in relaxed immobility; I squatted down beside him and found my attention equally divided between watching him and watching the trees. As the trees remained devoid of life, I concentrated on my companion. He sat there, clutching his spear upright in his large hands, and on his face was a look of eager expectancy, like that of a child at a pantomime before the curtain goes up. When he had appeared out of that dark little hut in Bafut, it seemed as though he had not only left behind his robes and trappings of state, but that he had also shed that regal air which had seemed so much part of his character. Here, crouching in this quiet, warm valley with his spear, he appeared to be just another hunter, his bright dark eyes fixed on the trees, waiting for the quarry he knew would come. But, as I looked at him, I realized that he was not just another hunter; there was something different about him which I could not place. It came to me what it was: any ordinary hunter would have crouched there, patient, a trifle bored, for he would have done the same thing so many times before. But the Fon waited, his eyes gleaming, a half-smile on his wide mouth, and I realized that he was thoroughly enjoying himself. I wondered how many times in the past he had become tired of his deferential councillors and his worshipping subjects, and felt his magnificent

robes to be hot and cumbersome and his pointed shoes cramp-
ing and hard. Then perhaps the urge had come to him to feel
the soft red earth under his bare feet and the wind on his naked
body, so that he would steal off to his hut, put on the clothes
of a hunter, and stride away over the hills, twirling his spear
and humming, pausing on the hilltops to admire the beautiful
country over which he ruled. I remembered the words he had
spoken to me only a short time before, 'If a man has hunting
for his eyes, his nose, and his blood, he never gets too old to go
to bush.' The Fon, I decided, was definitely one of that sort of
men. My meditations on the Fon's character were interrupted:
he leant forward and gripped my arm, pointing a long finger
at the trees.

'Dey done come,' he whispered, his face wreathed in smiles.

I followed the pointing of his finger, and for a moment I
could see nothing but a confused net of branches. Then something moved, and I saw the animal that we had been awaiting.

It came drifting through the tangled branches with all the
gentle, airy grace of a piece of thistledown. When it got nearer,
I discovered that it looked exactly like my idea of a leprechaun:
it was clad in a little fur coat of greenish-grey, and it had a long,
slender, furry tail. Its hands, which were pink, were large for
its size, and its fingers tremendously long and attenuated. Its
ears were large and the skin so fine that it was semi-transparent;
these ears seemed to have a life of their own, for they twisted
and turned independently, sometimes crumpling and folding
flat to the head as if they were a fan, at others standing up
pricked and straight like anaemic arum lilies. The face of the
little creature was dominated by a pair of tremendous dark
eyes, eyes that would have put any self-respecting owl to
shame. Moreover, the creature could twist its head round and
look over its back in much the same way that an owl does. It
ran to the tip of a slender branch that scarcely dipped beneath
its weight, and there it sat, clutching the bark with its long,
slender fingers, peering about with its great eyes and chirrup-
ing dimly to itself. It was, I knew, a galago, but it looked much
more like something out of a fairy tale.

It sat on the branch, twittering vaguely to itself, for about a

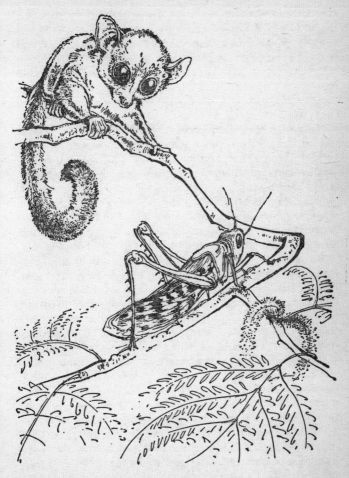

minute; then an astonishing thing happened. Quite suddenly the trees were full of galagos, galagos of every age and size, ranging from those little bigger than a walnut to adults that could have fitted themselves quite comfortably into an ordinary drinking-glass. They jumped from branch to branch, grasping the leaves and twigs with their large, thin hands, twittering softly to each other and gazing round them with the wide-eyed innocence of a troupe of cherubim. The baby ones, who seemed to be composed almost entirely of eyes, kept fairly close to their parents; occasionally they would sit up on their hind legs and hold up their tiny pink hands, fingers spread wide, as though in horror at the depravity they were seeing in the world of leaves around them.

One of these babies discovered, while I watched, that he was sitting on the same branch as a large and succulent locust. It was evening time, and the insect was drowsy and slow to realize its danger. Before it could do anything, the baby galago had flitted down the branch and grabbed it firmly round the middle. The locust woke up abruptly and decided that something must be done. It was a large insect, and was, in fact, almost as big as the baby galago; also it possessed a pair of long and muscular hind legs, and it started to kick out vigorously with them. It was a fascinating fight to watch: the galago clasped the locust desperately in his long fingers, and tried to bite it. Each time he tried to bite, the locust would give a terrific kick with its hind legs and knock its adversary off balance, so he would fall off the branch and hang underneath, suspended by his feet. When this had happened several times, I decided that the galago must have adhesive soles. And even when hanging upside down and being kicked in the stomach by a large locust, he maintained his expression of wide-eyed innocence.

The end of the fight was unexpected: when they were hanging upside down, the locust gave an extra hefty kick, and the galago's feet lost their grip, so that they fell through the leaves clasped together. As they tumbled earthwards, the galago loosened one hand from his grip round the locust's waist and grabbed a passing branch with the effortless ease of a trained acrobat. He hauled himself on to the branch and bit the locust's head off before the insect could recover sufficiently to continue the fight. Holding the decapitated but still kicking body in one hand, the galago stuffed the insect's head into his mouth and chewed it with evident enjoyment. Then he sat, clasping the twitching body in one hand and contemplated it with his head on one side, giving vent to shrill and excited screams of delight. When the corpse had ceased to move and the big hind legs had stiffened in death, the galago tore them off, one by one, and ate them. He looked ridiculously like a diminutive elderly gourmet, clasping in one hand the drumstick of some gigantic chicken.

Soon the valley was filled with shadow and it became difficult to see the galagos among the leaves, though we could hear their soft chittering. We rose from our cramped positions and made our way back up the hillside. At the top the Fon paused and gazed down at the woods below, smiling delightedly.

'Dat beef!' he chuckled, 'I like um too much. All time 'e make funny for me, an' I go laugh.'

'Na fine beef,' I said. 'How you call um?'

'For Bafut,' said the Fon, 'we call um Shilling.'

'You think sometimes my hunter men fit catch some?'

'To-morrow you go have some,' promised the Fon, but he would not tell me how they were to be captured, nor who was to do the capturing. We reached Bafut in the dusk, and when the Fon was respectably clothed once more he came and had a drink. As I said good night to him, I reminded him of his promise to get me some of the galagos.

'Yes, my friend, I no go forget,' he said. 'I go get you some Shilling.'

Four days passed, and I began to think that either the Fon had forgotten, or else the creatures were proving more difficult to capture than he had imagined. Then, on the fifth morning, my tea was brought in, and reposing on the tray was a small, highly-coloured raffia basket. I pulled off the lid and looked sleepily inside, and four pairs of enormous, liquid, innocent eyes peered up at me with expressions of gentle inquiry.

It was a basketful of Shillings from the Fon.

CHAPTER SEVEN

The Que-Fong-Goo

THE grassland country was populated by a rich variety of reptile life, and most of it seemed easily caught. In the lowland forests you very rarely saw a snake of any description, even if you searched for them. There *were* snakes there, of course, but I think that they were more widely dispersed, and probably most of the species were tree-dwellers, which made them much more difficult to see and to capture. In the mountains, however, the grass was alive with small rodents and frogs, and the patches of mountain forest filled with birds, so it was a paradise for snakes. There were great black spitting cobras, green mambas, slim tree-snakes with enormous, innocent-looking eyes, the multi-coloured Gaboon viper, with a forked rhino-like horn on its nose, and a host of others. As well as snakes, there were plenty of frogs and toads; the frogs ranged in size from the Hairy Frog down to tiny tree-frogs the size of an acorn, some spotted and streaked with such a dazzling array of colours that they looked more like delicious sweets than amphibians. The toads, on the whole, were fairly drab, but they made up for this by being decorated with strange clusters of warts and protuberances on their bodies, and an astonishing variety of colouring in their eyes.

But the commonest of the reptiles were the liza...
could be found everywhere; in the long herbage at the ...
scuttled fat skinks with stubby legs, fawn and silver and ...
in colour, and on the walls of the huts, in the road, and on ...
rocks the rainbow-coloured agamas pranced and nodded. Under the bark of trees or beneath stones you could find small geckos with great golden eyes, their bodies neatly and handsomely marked in chocolate and cream, and in the houses at night the ordinary house geckos, translucent and ghostly as pink pearls, paraded across the ceiling.

All these reptiles were brought in to me at one time or another by the local population. Sometimes it would be a snake tied insecurely to the end of a stick, or a calabash full of gulping frogs. Sometimes the capture would be carefully wrapped in the hunter's hat or shirt, or dangling on the end of a fine string. By these haphazard and dangerous methods such things as cobras, mambas, and Gaboon vipers would be brought to me, and although their captors knew their deadliness they handled them with an offhand carelessness that amazed me. As a rule, the African is no fool over snakes and prefers to regard every species as poisonous, just to be on the safe side, so to find the Bafutians treating them with such casualness was surprising, to say the least. I found it even more surprising when I discovered that the one reptile they all feared intensely was completely harmless.

I was out with the Bafut Beagles one day, and during the course of the hunt we came to a wide grassy valley about half a mile from the village. The Beagles had wandered off to set the nets, and while waiting for them I sat down in the grass to enjoy a cigarette. Suddenly my attention was attracted by a slight movement to my left, and on looking down I saw a reptile whose appearance made me gasp; hitherto I had been under the impression that the most colourful lizard in the grasslands was the agama, but, in comparison with the one that had crawled into view among the grass stems, the agama was as dull and colourless as a lump of putty. I sat there hardly daring to move, in case this wonderful creature dashed off into the herbage; as I remained quite still, it eventually decided that I was harmless, so slowly and luxuriously it slithered out into the sun and lay there contemplating me with its golden-flecked eyes. I could see that it was a skink of sorts, but one of the largest and most colourful skinks I had ever seen. It lay there quite still, basking in the early morning sun, so I had plenty of time to examine it.

Including its tail, it was about a foot in length and some two inches across the widest part of its body. It had a short, broad head and small but powerful legs. Its colouring and pattern were so dazzling and so intricate that it is almost impossible to describe. To begin with, the scales were large and very slightly raised, so that the whole creature looked as though it had been cleverly constructed out of mosaic. The throat was banded lengthwise with black and white, the top of the head was reddish-rust colour, while the cheeks, upper lip, and chin were bright brick red. The main body colour was a deep glossy black, against which the other colours showed up extremely well. Running from the angle of the jaw to the front legs were stripes of bright cherry red separated from each other by narrower bands composed of black-and-white scales. The tail and the outsides of the legs were spotted with white, the spots being fine and small on the legs, but so thickly distributed on the tail that in places they formed vertical bands. Its back was striped lengthwise in alternate stripes of black and canary yellow. As if that was not enough, the yellow stripes were broken in places by a series of pinkish scales. The whole reptile was bright and glossy, looking as though it had just been varnished and was still sticky.

As the skink and I sat there and watched each other I was busy trying to work out a plan for its capture. The butterfly net was some twenty feet away, but it might just as well have been in England for all the use it was, for I knew the skink would not lie there and allow me to trot over and fetch it. Behind him stretched a limitless jungle of long grass, and once he ran into that I knew he would disappear for good. Just then, to my dismay, I heard the Beagles returning. I knew I should have to do something quickly, as their approach would frighten the reptile. Slowly I rose to my feet, and the skink raised his head in alarm; as the first of the Beagles trotted through the grass, I flung myself desperately towards the skink. I had him at a slight disadvantage, for, having contemplated me in a motionless condition for a quarter of an hour, he had not expected me to launch myself through the air like a hawk. But my advantage was only temporary, for he recovered from his surprise quickly enough, and as I landed in the grass with a thump he scuttled to one side with great agility. I rolled over and made a wild grab at his rapidly retreating form, and as I did so the Beagle entered the clearing and saw what I was doing. Instead of leaping to my rescue, as I had expected, he uttered a prolonged shriek, jumped forward, and proceeded to drag me away from my quarry. The skink scuttled off into the dense tangle of grass and was lost; I shook off the Beagle's clutch on my arm and turned on him savagely.

'Bushman!' I snarled angrily. 'Na what foolish ting you do?'

'Masa,' said the Beagle, clicking his fingers in agitation, 'na bad, bad beef, dat ting. If 'e go bite Masa, Masa go die one time.'

With an effort I controlled my irritation. I had long ago found that, in spite of all arguments, the Africans clung tenaciously to their belief that some harmless species of reptile were deadly poisonous. So I resisted the temptation of telling the Beagle that he was an unmitigated idiot, and tried another line of argument instead.

'How you de call dis beef?' I asked.

'We call um Que-fong-goo, sah.'

'You say he get poison too much, eh?'

'Time no dere, Masa. Na bad beef.'

'All right, stupid man, you done forget that European get special medicine for dis kind of beef, eh? You done forget if dis beef go bite me I no go die, eh?'

'Eh! Masa, I done forget dis ting.'

'So you go run like woman, you de hollar and you de hold me so I go lose dis fine beef because you forget, eh?'

'Sorry, sah,' said the Beagle contritely.

I tapped his woolly skull with my finger.

'Next time, my friend,' I said sternly, 'you go tink with your brain before you go do dis kind of ting, you hear?'

'I hear, sah.'

When the other Beagles arrived on the scene, the incident was described to them, and there was much gasping and clicking of fingers.

'Wah!' said one of them admiringly. 'Masa no get fear. 'E done try for catch Que-fong-goo.'

'An' Uano done catch Masa,' said another, and they all laughed uproariously.

'Ay, Uano, you get lucky to-day. Sometime Masa go kill you for do dis stupid ting,' said another, and they all went off into fresh paroxysms of laughter at the thought of the Beagle having the temerity to stop me catching a specimen.

When they had recovered from the humour of the situation, I questioned them closely about the reptile. To my relief they assured me that it was fairly common in the grasslands and I should have plenty of opportunities of obtaining more specimens. They were all agreed, however, on the deadly properties of the skink. It was so poisonous, they assured me, that even if you so much as touched its body you immediately fell to the ground writhing in agony, and died within a few minutes. Then they asked me about the medicine I had to counteract this deadly creature, but I was suitably mysterious. I said if they found me a Que-fong-goo I would catch it and prove to them that I did not die writhing in agony. Cheered and intrigued by the thought of this grisly experiment (for none of them really believed in my medicine), they promised to do this. One of the Beagles said that he knew of a place where a great many such reptiles were to be found; he insisted that it was not very far distant, so we packed up the equipment and set off, the hunters chattering away to each other, presumably laying bets as to whether or not I could survive an encounter with a Que-fong-goo.

The Beagle eventually led us to a hillside about a mile away. The heavy mountain rains had stripped most of the red earth from the slope and left great sheets of grey rock exposed in its place. Occasional clefts in the rock had allowed a pocket of earth to form, and in these grew such plants as could draw nourishment from so small an area of soil. The sheets of rock were hemmed in by tall golden grass and a curious thistle-like plant with a pale buttercup-yellow head. The rock, lying exposed to the sun, was almost too hot to touch; the thin rubber soles of my shoes stuck to the surface as I walked across, so that I felt as though I was walking over a fly-paper. I began to wonder if this baking rock-face would not prove too much for even the most sun-loving of reptiles. Suddenly a flying streak of colour shot out of a clump of low growth across the shimmering rock, and disappeared into the sanctuary of the long grass and thistles.

'Que-fong-goo!' said the Bafut Beagles, stopping short and clutching their spears more tightly. Thinking that they would probably be more hindrance than help in any capture I might have to make, I told them to stay where they were and went ahead by myself. I had armed myself with a butterfly net, and as I cautiously approached the clumps of herbage that grew in the rock crevices I prodded them gently with the handle of the net to make sure there were no Que-fong-goos lurking inside. It was quite astonishing what even a small clump of grass would contain, and I disturbed innumerable large locusts, clouds of moths and gnats, a mass of brilliant butterflies, some beetles, and a few dragon-flies. I began to understand the attractions that this scorched and barren place might have for lizards.

Presently I struck lucky: on inserting the net handle into a clump of grass and wiggling it gently, I disturbed a Que-fong-goo. He slithered out of hiding and skimmed across the rough surface of the rock as smoothly as a stone on ice. I gave chase, but discovered almost immediately that a skink's idea of suitable country for sprinting was not mine. I caught my toe in a crack and fell flat on my face, and by the time I had picked myself up and recovered the net my quarry had disappeared. By now I was dripping with sweat, and the heat from the rock slabs was so great that any exertion made the blood pound in my head like a drum. The Beagles were standing at the edge of the long grass in a silent and fascinated group watching my progress. I wiped my face, clutched the net in one sticky hand and approached the next clump of grass doggedly. Here I was more careful; I edged the handle in among the grass-stalks and moved it to and fro very gently and slowly once or twice, and then withdrew it to see what would happen. I was rewarded by the sight of a Que-fong-goo, who stuck his head out of the undergrowth in a cautious manner to see what had caused the upheaval. Quickly I kicked the clump of grass behind him, and swept the net down as he ran out. The next moment I lifted the net triumphantly with the Que-fong-goo lashing furiously about in its folds. I pushed my hand inside the net and grabbed the reptile round the middle, and he retaliated by fastening his jaws on my thumb. Though his jaws were powerful, his teeth were minute, so his bite was quite painless and harmless. In order to keep him occupied, I let him chew away on my thumb, while I lifted him from the net. I held his dazzling beautiful body up aloft and waved it like a banner.

'Lookum!' I shouted to the Beagles, who were watching me open-mouthed. 'I done catch Que-fong-goo!'

As the Beagles were carrying the soft cloth bags I used to transport reptiles in, I left the net lying on the rocks and walked towards them, still clutching the skink in my hand. As one man, the Bafut Beagles dropped their spears and fled into the long grass like a herd of startled antelopes.

'What you de fear, eh?' I shouted. 'I go hold um tight for my hand, I no go let um run.'

'Masa, we de fear too much,' they replied in chorus, keeping a safe distance away in the long grass.

'Bring me bag for put dis beef,' I ordered sternly, mopping my brow.

'Masa we de fear . . . na bad beef dat,' came the cry again.

It became apparent that I should have to think of a fairly stiff argument, or else I should have to pursue my tribe of hunters all over the grasslands in my efforts to get a bag to put the skink in. I sat down at the edge of the long grass and glared at them.

'If someone no go bring me bag for put dis beef *one time*,' I proclaimed loudly and angrily, 'to-morrow I go get new hunter man. And, if de Fon go ask me why I go do dis ting, I go tell him I want hunter man who no get fear, I no want women.'

A silence descended upon the long grass while the Bafut Beagles decided whether it was better to face a Que-fong-goo in the hand, or a Fon at Bafut. After a short time the Que-fong-goo won, and they approached me slowly and reluctantly. One of them, still keeping a safe distance, threw me a bag to put my capture in, but before I put the skink inside it I thought a little demonstration would be a good thing.

'Lookum,' I said, holding the struggling lizard up for them to see. 'Now, you go watch fine and you see dis beef no get power for poison me.'

Holding the skink in one hand, I slowly brought the fore-finger of my other hand close to his nose; the reptile immediately gaped in a fearsome manner, and, amid cries of horror from the Beagles, I stuffed as much of my finger as I could into his mouth and let him chew on it. The Bafut Beagles stood rooted to the spot, watching with expressions of incredulous stupefaction as the reptile gnawed away at my finger, their eyes were wide, they held their breath and leant slightly forward with open mouths as they watched to see if the creature's bite would have any effect. After a few seconds the Que-fong-goo tired of biting ineffectually at my finger, and let go. I dropped him neatly into the bag and tied up the neck before turning to the hunters.

'You see?' I inquired. 'Dis beef done bit me, no be so?'

'Na so, sah,' came an awed whisper from the Beagles.

'All right: he done give me poison, eh? You tink sometime I go die, eh?'

'No, sah. If dat beef done bite Masa and Masa no die one time, den Masa no go die atall.'

'No, dis special medicine I done get,' I lied, shrugging with becoming modesty.

'Whah! Na so; Masa get fine medicine,' said the Beagles.

I had not gone through all this merely as a demonstration of the white man's superiority over the black; the true reason for this little charade was that I dearly wanted a great many

Que-fong-goos and I knew that I should not obtain them unless I had the help and co-operation of the Beagles. In order to get this, I had to overcome their fear, and the only way I could do this was by showing them that my mythical medicine was more than a match for the deadly bite of the Que-fong-goo. At some future date, I thought, I would provide them with a quantity of innocuous liquid disguised as the medicine in question, and, armed with this elixir, they would sally forth and return with sackfuls of glittering Que-fong-goos.

On the way back to Bafut I strutted along, proudly carrying my precious skink and feeling very pleased with myself for having devised such a cunning scheme for obtaining more of the lovely reptiles. Behind me the Beagles trotted in silence, still gazing at me with awed expressions. Each time we passed someone on the path they would give a rapid *résumé* of my powers, and I would hear gasps of surprise and horror as the tale was told, slightly embellished with each repetition, I have no doubt. When we reached the villa, and I had my skink nicely housed in a large box, I gathered the Beagles together and made them a little speech. I pointed out that, as they had seen with their own eyes, my medicine was sufficient protection against the bites of Que-fong-goos. They all nodded vigorously. Therefore, I went on, as I wanted a great many specimens of the reptile, I proposed to supply them with the magic potion the next day, and thus armed they would be able to go out and hunt Que-fong-goos for me. Then I beamed at them complacently, waiting for the cries of delight I expected. None came; instead the Beagles stood there looking extremely glum and twiddling their toes in the dust.

'Well,' I inquired after a long pause, 'you no agree?'

'No, Masa,' they mumbled.

'Why you no agree? You no savvay dat I go give you dis special medicine, eh? Why you de fear?'

They scratched their heads, shuffled their feet, glanced helplessly at each other, and then one of them eventually plucked up the courage to speak.

'Masa,' he said, having cleared his throat several times, 'dis medicine you done get na fine one. We savvay dis ting. We don see dis beef bite Masa time no dere, and Masa no die.'

'Well?'

'Dis medicine, Masa, na juju for white man. No be juju for black man. For Masa na good ting dis medicine, but for we no be good ting.'

For half an hour I argued, pleaded, and cajoled them. They were polite but firm; the medicine was fine for whites, but it would not work with black people. That was their belief and they were sticking to it. I tried every argument I could think of to make them change their minds, but it was no use. At last, thoroughly irritated by the failure of my little scheme, I dismissed the Beagles and stalked off to have my meal.

Later that evening the Fon turned up, accompanied by five council members and a bottle of gin. We sat on the moonlit veranda for half an hour or so, discussing various subjects in a desultory fashion, and then the Fon hitched his chair closer to mine and leant forward, giving me his wide and engaging grin that lit up his whole face.

'Some man done tell me dat you done catch Que-fong-goo,' he said. 'Dis man speak true?'

'Na so,' I nodded, 'na fine beef dat.'

'Dis man done say you catch dis beef with your hand,' said the Fon. 'I tink sometime dis man tell me lie, eh? Dis na bad beef, dis Que-fong-goo; you no fit catch um with you hand, eh? 'E go kill you one time, no be so?'

'No,' I said firmly, 'dis man no tell lie. I done catch dis beef with my hand.'

The council members let out their breath with a hiss at this information, and the Fon sat back and regarded me wide-eyed.

'An when you done catch um what 'e done do?' asked the Fon at last.

'He done bite me.'

'Whaaaaa!' said the Fon and the council members in unison.

'He done bite me here,' I said, holding out my hand, and the Fon shied away as though I had pointed a gun at him. He and the council members examined my finger from a safe distance, chattering eagerly to each other.

'Why you no die?' asked the Fon presently.

'Die?' I asked, frowning. 'Why I go die?'

'Na bad beef dis ting,' said the Fon excitedly. ''E de bite too much. If black man go hold him 'e go die one time. Why you never die, my friend?'

'Oh, I get special medicine for dis ting,' I said airily.

A chorus of 'Ahhs!' came from my audience.

'Na European medicine dis?' asked the Fon.

'Yes. You like I go show you?'

'Yes, yes, na foine!' he said eagerly.

They sat there silent and expectant while I went and fetched my small medicine chest; from it I extracted a packet of boracic powder, and spread a little on the palm of my hand. They all craned eagerly forward to see it. I filled a glass of water, mixed in the powder and then rubbed the result on my hands.

'There!' I said, spreading my hands out like a conjurer.

'Now Que-fong-goo no fit kill me.'

I walked over to the skink box, opened it, and turned round holding the beast in my hands. There was a fluttering of robes and the council members fled to the other end of the veranda in a disorderly stampede. The Fon remained rooted to his chair, a look of disgust and fright on his face as I walked towards him. I stopped in front of him and held out the reptile, who was busily trying to amputate my finger.

'Look . . . you see?' I said; 'dis beef no fit kill me.'

The Fon's breath escaped in a prolonged 'Aieeeeeee!' of astonishment as he watched the lizard. Presently he tore his fascinated eyes away from it and looked up at me.

'Dis medicine,' he said hoarsely, ''e good for black man?'

'Na fine for black man.'

'Black man no go die?'

'Atall, my friend.'

The Fon sat back and gazed at me in wonder.

'Wha!' he said at last, 'na fine ting dis.'

'You like you go try dis medicine?' I asked casually.

'Er . . . er . . . yes, yes, na foine,' said the Fon nervously.

Before he could change his mind, I put the skink back in the box, and then prepared some more of the boracic mixture. I showed the Fon how to rub it on his enormous hands, and he massaged away for a long time. Then I brought the box, pulled out the skink, and held it out for him.

It was a tense moment; the ring of council members watched with bated breath and screwed-up countenances while the Fon licked his lips, put out his hand towards the skink, drew it back nervously, and then reached out again. There was a moment's suspense as his hand lowered over the highly-coloured reptile, then he drew a deep breath and grabbed the beast firmly round the waist.

'Ahhh!' hissed the council members.

'Wheee! I done hold um,' yelped the Fon, clutching the unfortunate skink so tightly that I feared for its life.

'Hold um softly,' I begged. 'You go kill um if you hold um tight.'

But the Fon, paralysed by a mixture of fright and pleasure at his own daring, could only sit there glaring at the skink in his hand and muttering, 'I done hold um ... I done hold um ...' until I was forced to prise the unfortunate skink loose and return it to its box.

The Fon examined his hands, and then looked up at me with an expression of child-like delight on his face. The council members were chattering away to each other. The Fon waved his hands at me and started to laugh. He laughed and laughed and laughed, slapping his thighs, doubling up in his chair, coughing and spluttering, while the tears ran down his face. It was so infectious that I started to laugh as well, and soon the councillors joined in. We sat there stamping our feet, laughing as though we would never stop until some of the councillors rolled on the floor and fought for breath, and the Fon lay back weakly in his chair shaken by huge gusts of mirth.

'Why you de laugh?' I spluttered at last.

'Na funny ting,' said the Fon, shaken with fresh laughter, 'for long time, ever since I be picken, I done fear dis beef. Wah! I done fear um too much. Now you give me medicine and I no de fear any more.'

He leant back in his chair and sobbed with mirth at the thought.

'Que-fong-goo, your time done pass; I no go fear you again,' he gurgled.

Later, still aching from our laughter, we finished our drinks, and the Fon went back to his own villa, carefully clutching a small packet of boracic powder. I had warned him that although the medicine could be used with success against Que-fong-goos, agamas, and geckos, it could not, in any circumstances, be used to guard against the bite of snakes. As I had hoped, the story that the Fon had picked up a Que-fong-goo after having been immunized by my medicine, and that he had survived the encounter, was common gossip the next day. In the afternoon the Bafut Beagles turned up, and stood grinning at me disarmingly.

'Whatee?' I asked coldly.

'Masa,' said the Beagles, 'give us dat medicine you done give for Fon, and we go hunt Que-fong-goos for Masa.'

That evening I had two boxes full of the beautiful grassland skinks, and the Bafut Beagles were drinking corn beer, surrounded by an admiring crowd of Bafutians, while they recounted the story of the day's hunt, with, I have no doubt, suitable embellishments. While I listened to them, I sat on the veranda and wrote a note to the nearest U.A.C. stores, asking them to send me another packet of boracic. I felt that it might come in useful.

CHAPTER EIGHT

The Typhlops in Disguise

AFTER a few weeks the number of people who brought me specimens dwindled to a steady daily trickle. This was because I had, by this time, obtained enough of the commoner species of animals, and I was refusing to buy any more of them. The veranda outside my bedroom was piled high with a strange variety of cages, containing the most fantastically assorted collection of mammals, birds, and reptiles, and my mornings and the better part of my evenings were devoted to their care. My days were full, but never dull; apart from cleaning and feeding the collection, there was endless enjoyment to be got from watching the habits of my specimens and their reaction to captivity and to myself. Then there was the life of Bafut. Working on the veranda I was in an elevated vantage point that commanded an excellent view of the road and the Fon's courtyard and houses. Peering through the tattered fringe of bougainvillaea, I could watch the movements of the Fon's numerous wives, offspring, and councillors, and the constant comings and goings of the Bafut population on the road. From the veranda I observed many a scene enacted below me, and by reaching out a hand for my field-glasses I could bring the actors so close that every slight change of expression on their faces could be noticed.

One evening I saw a slim, good-looking girl walk down the road; she was meandering, dragging her feet, as though waiting for someone to catch up with her. I was just about to call a greeting to her as she passed beneath the house when I saw a powerful young man come trotting up behind her, his face distorted into a ferocious scowl. He called out sharply, and the girl paused, then turned round with an expression of sulky insolence on her handsome face, which the young man obviously found very irritating. He halted in front of her and started to talk in a loud and angry voice, gesturing fiercely with his arms, his eyes and teeth flashing in his dark face. The girl stood without movement, a faint, rather sneering smile on her lips. Then a third actor joined the scene: an old woman came scuttling down the road, screaming at the top of her voice and waving a long bamboo. The man took no notice of the newcomer, but continued his rather one-sided argument with the girl. The old woman danced round the two of them, brandishing her bamboo, screeching shrilly, her flat and wrinkled dugs flapping up and down on her chest as she moved. The more she screeched the louder the man shouted, and the more he shouted the more sullen became the girl's expression. Suddenly the old woman whirled round on one leg like a dervish and struck the man across the shoulders with her bamboo. The only notice he took of this assault was to reach out a long, muscular arm, twitch the stick from the old woman's hand, and fling it high into the air so that it fell over the red brick wall into the great courtyard. The old woman stood nonplussed for a moment, then she danced up behind the young man and kicked him hard in the behind. He took no notice whatsoever, but continued to shout at the girl, his gestures getting wilder and wilder. All at once the girl snarled some reply at him and spat accurately on to his feet.

The young man up till then had obviously been adopting a non-belligerent attitude, and he had, I felt, been getting the worst of things; the women, I decided, were taking an unfair advantage of him. However, having his feet spat upon was apparently the last straw; he stood for a moment open-mouthed at such a treacherous attack, and then with a roar of rage he leapt forward, grasped the girl round the throat with one hand while boxing her ears soundly with the other, and finally gave her a push so that she fell to the ground. The old woman was quite overcome by this action, falling flat on her back into the ditch and indulging in the finest fit of hysterics I have ever seen. Rolling from side to side and patting her mouth, she gave vent to prolonged Red Indian hoots of the most blood-curdling quality. Occasionally, she would break off these noises to scream. The girl lay in the red dust, sobbing bitterly; the man took no notice of the old lady, but squatted down beside the girl and appeared to be pleading with her. After a while the girl looked up and gave a watery smile, whereupon the young man sprang to his feet, grabbed her by the wrist and they set off down the road, leaving the old woman still rolling and hooting in the ditch.

I was, quite frankly, puzzled by the whole affair. What had it all been about? Was the girl the man's wife, and had she been unfaithful to him, and had he found out? But what then was the reason for the old woman's presence? Perhaps the girl had stolen something from the man? Or, more likely, the girl and the old woman had been practising juju on him, and he had found out? Juju, I thought; that must be the explanation. The girl, tiring of her young husband, had tried to poison him by mixing chopped-up leopard whiskers with his food – leopard whiskers which she had obtained from the old woman, who was, of course, a well-known local witch. But the husband had become suspicious, and the girl had fled to the witch for protection. The husband had followed the girl, and the witch (who felt some sort of obligation towards her customers) had followed them both to try to sort things out. I had just worked this theory out into a form that would have been acceptable to the *Wide World Magazine*, when I looked over the edge of the veranda and saw Jacob below peering through the hedge at the old woman, who was still rolling in the ditch and making noises reminiscent of Clapham Junction.

'Jacob,' I called, 'na whatee all dat palaver?'

Jacob looked up and gave a throaty chuckle.

'Dis ole woman, sah, she be mammy for dat picken woman.

Dat picken woman be wife for dat man. Dat man 'e done go
for bush all day, an' when 'e done come back 'e find 'e wife
never make him food. 'E belly de cry out, an' de man angry too
much, so he like beat 'e wife. De wife 'e run, de man 'e run,
for beat 'e wife, an' de ole woman 'e run for beat dis man.'

I was bitterly disappointed; I felt that Africa, the dark and
mysterious continent, had let me down. Instead of my juicy
intrigue, my witches and magic potions full of leopard
whiskers, I had been witnessing an ordinary domestic upheaval with the usual ingredients of an erring wife, a hungry
husband, an uncooked dinner, and an interfering mother-in-
law. I turned my attention back to the collection, feeling
distinctly cheated. It was the mother-in-law, I think, that
rankled most.

Not long after this there was another upheaval on and
around the veranda, in which I played the chief part, but it was
not until long afterwards that I was able to appreciate its
humour. It was a beautiful evening, and in the west shoals of
narrow, puffy clouds were assembling for what was obviously
going to be a glorious sunset.

I had just finished a well-earned cup of tea, and was sitting
on the top step in the late sunlight trying to teach an incredibly stupid baby squirrel how to suck milk from a blob
of cotton wool on the end of a matchstick. Pausing for a
moment in this nerve-racking work, I saw a fat and elderly
woman waddling down the road. She was wearing the briefest
of loin-cloths, and was smoking a long, slender black pipe.
On top of her grey, cropped hair was perched a tiny calabash.
When she reached the bottom step, she knocked out her pipe
and hung it carefully from the cord round her ample waist,
before starting to climb towards the veranda.

'Iseeya, Mammy,' I called.

She stopped and grinned up at me.

'Iseeya, Masa,' she replied, and then continued to heave her
body from step to step, panting and wheezing with the exertion. When she reached me, she placed the calabash at my feet,
and then leant her bulk against the wall, gasping for breath.

'You done tire, Mammy?' I asked.

'Wah! Masa, I get fat too much,' she explained.

'Fat!' I said in shocked tones; 'you no get fat, Mammy. You no get fat pass me.'

She chuckled richly, and her gigantic body quivered.

'No, Masa, you go fun with me.'

'No, Mammy, I speak true, you be small woman.'

She fell back against the wall, convulsed with laughter at the thought of being called a small woman, her vast stomach and breasts heaving. Presently, when she had recovered from the joke, she gestured at the calabash.

'I done bring beef for you, Masa.'

'Na what kind of beef?'

'Na snake, Masa.'

I unplugged the calabash and peered inside. Coiled up in the bottom was a thin, brown snake about eight inches long. I recognized it as a typhlops, a species of blind snake which spends its life burrowing underground. It resembles the English slow-worm in appearance, and is quite harmless. I already had a box full of these reptiles, but I liked my fat girl friend so much that I did not want to disappoint her by refusing it.

'How much you want for dis beef, Mammy?' I asked.

'Eh, Masa go pay me how 'e tink.'

'Snake no get wound?'

'No, Masa, atall.'

I turned the calabash upside down and the snake fell out on to the smooth concrete. The woman moved to the other end of the veranda with a speed that was amazing for one so huge.

''E go bite you Masa,' she called warningly.

Jacob, who had appeared to see what was going on, gave the woman a withering look at this remark.

'You no savvay Masa no get fear for dis ting?' he asked. 'Masa get special juju so dis kind of snake no go chop 'e.'

'Ah, na so?' said the woman.

I leant forward and picked up the typhlops in my hand, so that I could examine it closely to make sure it was unhurt. I gripped its body gently between my thumb and forefinger, and it twisted itself round my finger. As I looked at it, I noticed a curious thing: it possessed a pair of large and glittering eyes, a thing which no typhlops ever possessed. Foolishly, rather startled by my discovery, I still held the reptile loosely in my hand, and spoke to Jacob.

'Jacob, look, dis snake 'e get eye,' I said.

As I spoke, I suddenly realized that I was holding loosely in my hand not a harmless typhlops but some unidentified snake of unknown potentialities. Before I could open my hand and drop it, the snake twisted round smoothly and buried a fang in the ball of my thumb.

Off-hand I can never remember receiving quite such a shock. The bite itself was nothing – like the prick of a pin, followed by a slight burning sensation, rather similar to a wasp sting. I dropped the snake with alacrity, and squeezed my thumb as hard as I could, so that the blood oozed out of the wound, and as I squeezed I remembered three things. First, there was no snake-bite serum in the Cameroons; secondly, the nearest doctor was some thirty miles away; thirdly, I had no means of getting to him. These thoughts did not make me feel any happier, and I sucked vigorously at the bite, still holding the base of my thumb as tightly as I could. Looking about, I found that Jacob had vanished, and I was just about to utter a roar of rage, when he came scurrying back on to the veranda, carrying in one hand a razor blade, and in the other a couple of ties. Under my frenzied directions, he tied the latter round my wrist and forearm as tightly as he could, and then, with a curious gesture, he handed me the razor blade.

I had never realized before quite how much determination it requires to slash yourself with a razor blade, nor had I realized quite how sharp a razor blade could be. After an awful moment's hesitation, I slashed at my hand, and then found I had given myself a nasty and unnecessary cut about half an inch away from the bite, in a place where it could be of no possible use.

I tried again, with much the same result, and I thought gloomily that if I did not die of the bite, I would probably bleed to death as a result of my own first aid. I thought vindictively of all those books I had read that gave tips on how to deal with snake-bite. All of them, without exception, told you how to make an incision across the bite to the full depth of the fang punctures. It's easy enough to write that sort of thing, but it is quite a different matter to put it into practice successfully when the thumb you are slitting open is your own. There was only one thing to be done, unless I wanted to go on hacking my hand about in the hope of hitting the bite sooner or later. I placed the blade carefully on the ball of my thumb and, gritting my teeth, I pressed and pulled as hard as I could. This was successful, and the blood flowed freely in all directions. The next thing to do, I remembered, was to use permanganate of potash, so I sprinkled some crystals into the gaping wound, and wrapped my hand in a clean handkerchief. By now my hand, wrist, and the glands in my armpit were considerably swollen, and I was getting shooting pains in my thumb, though whether this was due to the bite or to my surgery, I could not tell.

'Masa go for doctor?' asked Jacob, staring at my hand.

'How I go for doctor,' I asked irritably; 'we no get car for dis place. You tink sometimes I go walk?'

'Masa go ask de Fon for 'e kitcar,' suggested Jacob.

'Kitcar?' I repeated, hope dawning, 'de Fon get kitcar?'

'Yes, sah.'

'Go ask him den . . . one time.'

Jacob galloped down the steps and across the great courtyard, while I paced up and down on the balcony. Suddenly I remembered that in my bedroom reposed a large and untouched bottle of French brandy, and I sped inside in search of it. I had just managed to pull out the cork when I recalled that all the books on snake-bite were adamant when it came to the point of spirits. On no account, they all stated, must spirits be taken by anyone suffering from snake-bite; apparently they accelerated the heart action and did all sorts of other strange things to you. For a moment I paused, the bottle clutched in one hand; then I decided that if I were going to die I might as well die happy, and I raised the bottle and drank. Warmed and encouraged, I trotted out on to the veranda again, carrying the bottle with me.

A large crowd of people, headed by Jacob and the Fon, were

hurrying across the courtyard. They went over to a big hut, and the Fon threw open the door and the crowd poured inside, to reappear almost immediately pushing in front of them an ancient and battered kitcar. They trundled this out through the archway and into the road, and there the Fon left them and hurried up the steps followed by Jacob.

'My friend,' gasped the Fon, 'na bad palaver dis!'

'Na so,' I admitted.

'Your boy done tell me you no get European medicine for dis kind of bite. Na so?'

'Yes, na so. Sometime doctor done get medicine, I no savvay.'

'By God power 'e go give you medicine,' said the Fon piously.

'You go drink with me?' I asked, waving the bottle of brandy.

'Yes, yes,' said the Fon, brightening, 'we go drink. Drink na good medicine for dis kind of ting.'

Jacob brought glasses and I poured out a liberal measure for us both. Then we went to the top of the steps to see what progress was being made with the preparation of the ambulance.

The kitcar had reposed inside the hut for such a great length of time that its innards seemed to have seized up. Under the driver's gentle ministrations the engine coughed vigorously several times and then ceased. The large crowd round the vehicle clustered closer, all shouting instructions to him, while he leant out of the window and abused them roundly. This went on for some time, and then the driver climbed out and tried to crank her up. This was even less successful, and when he had exhausted himself, he handed the crank to a councillor and went and sat on the running-board for a rest. The councillor hitched up his robes and struggled manfully with the crank, but was unable to rouse the engine to life.

The crowd, which now numbered about fifty people, all clamoured for a turn, so the councillor handed the job over to them and joined the driver on the running-board. A disgraceful fight broke out among the crowd as to who would have first turn, and everyone was shouting and pushing and

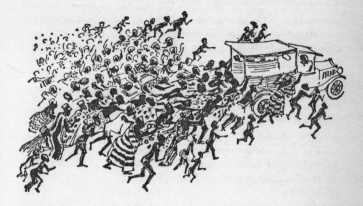

snatching the crank from one another. The uproar attracted
the attention of the Fon, and he drained his glass and stalked
over to the veranda rail, scowling angrily. He leant over and
glared down at the road.

'Wah!' he roared suddenly. 'Start dat motor!'

The crowd fell silent, and all turned to look up at the
veranda, while the driver and council member jumped off
the running-board and rushed round to the front of the car
with an amazing display of enthusiasm. This was somewhat
spoilt by the fact that when they did arrive there, the crank was
missing. Uproar started again, with everyone accusing everyone else of having lost it. It was found eventually, and the two
of them made several more ineffectual attempts to get the
engine started.

By now I was beginning to feel rather ill and not at all brave.
My hand and forearm had swollen considerably, and were in-
flamed and painful. I was also getting shooting pains across
my shoulders, and my hand felt as though it was grasping a
red-hot coal.

It would take me about an hour to reach the doctor, I
thought, and if the kitcar did not start soon, there would be
little point in going at all. The driver, having nearly ruptured
himself in his efforts to crank, was suddenly struck by a

brilliant idea. They would push the car. He explained his idea
to the crowd, and it was greeted with exclamations of delight
and acclamation. The driver got in and the crowd swarmed
round behind the kitcar and began to push. Grunting rhythmically, they pushed the kitcar slowly down the road, round
the corner, and out of sight.

'Soon 'e go start,' smiled the Fon encouragingly, pouring
me some more brandy, 'den you go reach doctor one time.'

'You tink 'e go start?' I asked sceptically.

'Yes, yes, ma friend,' said the Fon, looking hurt; 'na my
kitcar dis, na foine one. 'E go start small time, no go fear.'

Presently we heard the grunting again, and, on looking over
the veranda rail, we saw the kitcar appear round the corner,
still being propelled by what seemed to be the entire population of Bafut. It crept towards us like a snail, and then, just as
it reached the bottom step, the engine gave a couple of pre-
liminary hiccoughs and then roared into life. The crowd
screamed with delight and began to caper about in the road.

''E done start,' explained the Fon proudly, in case I had
missed the point of the celebrations.

The driver manoeuvred the car through the archway into
the courtyard, turned her round, and swept out on to the road
again, impatiently tootling his horn and narrowly missing his
erstwhile helpers. The Fon and I drained our glasses and then
marched down the seventy-five steps. At the bottom the Fon
clasped me to his bosom and gazed earnestly into my face. It
was obvious that he wanted to say something that would
encourage and sustain me on my journey. He thought deeply
for a moment.

'My friend,' he said at last, 'if you go die I get sorry too
much.'

Not daring to trust my voice, I clasped his hand in what I
hoped was a suitably affected manner, climbed into the kitcar
and we were off, bouncing and jerking down the road, leaving
the Fon and his subjects enveloped in a large cloud of red dust.

Three-quarters of an hour later we drew up outside the
doctor's house with an impressive squealing of brakes. The
doctor was standing outside gloomily surveying a flower-bed.

He looked at me in surprise when I appeared, and then, coming forward to greet me, he peered closely into my face.

'What have you been bitten by?' he inquired.

'How did you know I'd been bitten?' I asked, rather startled by this rapid diagnosis.

'Your pupils are tremendously distended,' explained the doctor with professional relish. 'What was it?'

'A snake. I don't know what kind, but it hurts like hell. I don't suppose there was really much use in my coming in to you. There's no serum to be had, is there?'

'Well!' he said in a pleased tone of voice. 'Isn't that a strange thing? Last time I was on leave I got some serum. Thought it might come in useful. It's been sitting in the fridge for the last six months.'

'Well, thank heaven for that.'

'Come into the house, my dear fellow. I shall be most interested to see if it works.'

'So shall I,' I admitted.

We went into the house, and I sat down in a chair while the doctor and his wife busied themselves with methylated spirits, hypodermic needles, and the other accoutrements necessary for the operation. Then the doctor gave me three injections in the thumb, as near to the bite as was possible, and a couple more in my arm. These hurt me considerably more than the original bite had done.

'Made you feel a bit rocky?' inquired the doctor cheerfully, feeling my pulse.

'They've made me feel bloody,' I said bitterly.

'What you need is a good stiff whisky.'

'I thought one wasn't allowed spirits?'

'Oh, yes. It won't hurt you,' he said, and poured me out a liberal glassful. I can never remember a drink tasting so good.

'And now,' the doctor went on, 'you're to spend the night in the spare room. I want you in bed in five minutes. You can have a bath if you feel like it.'

'Can't I go back to Bafut?' I asked. 'I've got all my animals there, and there's no one really competent to look after them.'

'You're in no state to go back to Bafut, or to look after

animals,' he said firmly. 'Now no arguments, into bed. You
can go back in the morning, if I think you're well enough.'

To my surprise, I slept soundly, and when I awoke the next
day I felt extremely well, though my arm was still swollen and
mildly painful. I had breakfast in bed, and then the doctor
came to have a look at me.

'How d'you feel?' he asked.

'Fine. I'm feeling so well that I'm beginning to think the
snake must have been harmless.'

'No, it was poisonous all right. You said it only got you
with one fang, and you probably dropped it so quickly that it
didn't have time to inject the full shot of venom. If it had, it
might have been another story.'

'Can I go back to Bafut?'

'Well, yes, if you feel up to it, but I shouldn't think that
arm will be up to much for a day or two. Anyway, if it worries
you, come in and see me.'

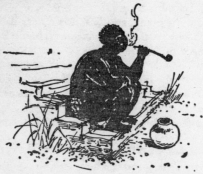

Spurred on by the thought of my precious collection waiting at Bafut, uncleaned and unfed, I goaded the unfortunate
driver so that he got us back in record time. As we drew up in
the road below the villa, I saw a figure seated on the bottom
step. It was my fat girl friend of the day before.

'Iseeya, Mammy,' I said, as I stepped down into the road.

'Iseeya, Masa,' she replied, hoisting herself to her feet and
waddling towards me.

'Na what you de want?' I asked, for I was impatient to get up to my animals.

'Masa done forget?' she inquired, surprised.

'Forget what, Mammy?'

'Eh, Masa!' she said accusingly, 'Masa never pay me for dat fine snake I done bring.'

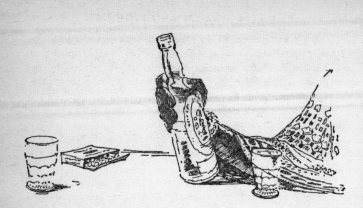

CHAPTER NINE

The Fon and the Golden Cat

MY stay in Bafut eventually drew to a close. I had collected a vast quantity of animal life, and it was time to take it all back to the base camp, where it could be re-caged and got ready for the voyage. Reluctantly I informed all the hunters that I would be leaving in a week, so that they would not bring in any specimens after I had left. I ordered the lorry, and sent a note to Smith, telling him to expect me. The Fon, when he heard the news, came flying over, clasping a bottle of gin, and did his best to persuade me to stay. But, as I explained to him, I could not stay any longer, much as I would like to do so; our return passages were booked, and that meant the whole collection had to be ready to move down country on the prescribed date. If there was any hitch we would miss the ship, and we might not be able to get another one for a couple of months, a delay which the trip's budget was not designed to cope with.

'Ah! my friend, I sorry too much you go,' said the Fon, pouring gin into my glass with the gay abandon of a fountain.

'I sorry too much as well,' I said with truth; 'but I no get chance for stay Bafut any more.'

'You go remember Bafut,' said the Fon, pointing a long finger at me; 'you go remember Bafut fine. Na for Bafut you done get plenty fine beef, no be so?'

'Na so,' I said, pointing at my vast piles of cages; 'I done get beef too much for Bafut.'

The Fon nodded benignly. Then he leant forward and clasped my hand.

'When you go for your country, sometime you go tell your people de Fon of Bafut na your friend, an 'e done get you all dis fine beef, eh?'

'I go tell um all,' I promised, 'and I go tell um dat de Fon be fine hunter man, better pass all hunter for Cameroons.'

'Foine, foine!' said the Fon delightedly.

'Na one beef I never get for here,' I said; 'I sorry too much.'

'Na whatee, my friend?' he asked, leaning forward anxiously.

'Na dat big bush cat dat get skin like gold and mark-mark for 'e belly. I done show you photograph, you remember?'

'Ah! Dat beef!' he said; 'you speak true. Dat beef you never get yet.'

He relapsed into a gloomy silence and scowled at the gin bottle. I wondered if perhaps reminding him of this gap in my collection had not been a little tactless. The animal to which I was referring was the Golden Cat, one of the smaller, but one of the most beautiful, members of the cat family to be found in that part of Africa. I knew that it was reasonably common around Bafut, but the hunters treated it with more respect than they showed for the Serval and the Leopard, both of which were considerably bigger. Whenever I had shown pictures of the beast to the hunters they had chuckled and shaken their heads over it, and assured me that it was extremely difficult to catch, that it was 'fierce too much' and that it 'get plenty clever'. In vain I had offered large rewards, not only for the animal's capture, but even for news of its whereabouts. With slightly less than a week to go before I left, I had resigned myself to not being able to add a Golden Cat to the collection.

The Fon sat back in his chair with a twinkle in his eye, and grinned at me infectiously.

'I go get you dat beef,' he said, nodding portentously.

'But, my friend, in five days I go leave Bafut. How you go catch dis beef in five days?'

'I go catch um,' said the Fon firmly. 'Wait small time you go see. I go get you dat beef.'

He refused to tell me by what methods he was going to bring about this miracle, but he was so sure of himself that I began to wonder if he really would be able to get me one of these creatures. When, however, the day before my departure dawned and there was no sign of any Golden Cat, I gave up all hope. In his enthusiasm, the Fon had made a promise which he could not fulfil.

It was a sombre, overcast day, for up there in the mountains the rainy season started earlier than in the lowlands. The low, fast-moving clouds, grey as slate, the thin drizzle of rain, and the occasional shudder of thunder in the distant mountain ranges, none of these things helped to make me feel any the less depressed at the thought of leaving Bafut. I had grown very fond of this silent grassland world, and of the people who lived there. The Fon I had come to admire and like, and I felt genuinely sorry at the thought of saying good-bye to him, for he had been an amusing and charming companion.

About four o'clock the fine drizzle turned into a steady downpour that blurred the landscape, drummed and rattled on the roof of the villa and the fronds of the palm trees nearby, turned the red earth of the great courtyard into a shimmering sea of blood-red clay freckled with pockmarks of the falling rain. I had finished my cleaning and feeding of the collection, and I wandered moodily up and down the veranda, watching the rain beat and bruise the scarlet bougainvillaea flowers against the brickwork. My luggage was packed, the cages were stacked and ready for loading into the lorry. I could think of nothing to do, and I did not fancy venturing out into the icy downpour.

Glancing down at the road, I saw a man appear at a trot, slipping and sliding in the mud, carrying on his back a large sack. Hoping that he was bringing me some rare specimen to lighten my gloom, I watched his approach eagerly, but to my

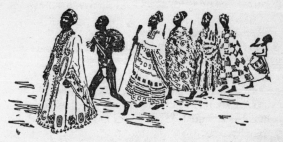

annoyance he turned off under the archway and splashed his way across the great courtyard and disappeared through the arched door leading to the Fon's quarters. Shortly after he had vanished, a loud uproar broke out near the Fon's small villa, but it died down after some minutes and all I could hear was the rain. I went and drank my tea in solitary state, and then finished feeding all the nocturnal creatures; they all looked a trifle surprised, for I did not feed them as early as that as a rule, but as the Fon was coming over to spend the evening I wanted to have everything done before he arrived. By the time I had finished my work the rain had died away to a fine, mist-like drizzle, and there were breaks appearing in the low-flying grey clouds through which the sky shone a pale and limpid blue. Within an hour the clouds had dispersed altogether, and the sky was smooth and clear and full of evening sunlight. A small drum started to beat over near the Fon's house, and the sound gradually grew louder. The door into the courtyard opened and a small procession marched through. First came the Fon, dressed in the most magnificent scarlet-and-white robes, striding delicately through the shining puddles. Following him came the strange man I had seen in the rain, still with the sack on his back. Behind him were four council members, and at the end of the procession trotted a small boy in white robes and minute skull-cap, beating importantly on a little drum. The Fon was obviously coming to pay me his last visit in some style. I went down the steps to meet him. He halted in front of me and put his hands on my shoulders, staring into my face with a most impressive sternness.

'My friend,' he said slowly and solemnly, 'I done get something for you.'

'Na whatee?' I asked.

The Fon flung back his trailing sleeves with a regal gesture, and pointed at the man with the sack.

'Bushcat!' he said.

For a moment I was puzzled, and then suddenly I remembered the creature he had promised to get for me.

'Bushcat? Dat kind I de want too much?' I asked, hardly daring to believe it.

The Fon nodded with the quiet satisfaction of one who has done a job well.

'Let me look um,' I said excitedly; 'quick, open dat bag.'

The man placed the sack on the ground in front of me, and I, forgetful of the clean trousers I had put on in the Fon's honour, went down on my knees in the mud and struggled with the tough cord that bound the neck of the sack. The Fon stood by, beaming down at me like a benevolent Santa Claus. The cord was wet and tight, and as I tugged and pulled at it there arose from the interior of the sack a weird and ferocious cry: it started as a rumbling moan, and as it became louder it developed into a yarring scream with such a malevolent undertone that it sent a chill up my spine. The hunter, the councillors and the boy with the drum all retreated several paces.

'Careful, Masa,' the hunter warned; 'na bad beef dat. 'E get power too much.'

'You done get rope for 'e foot?' I asked, and he nodded.

I unwound the last bit of cord, and then slowly opened the sack and peered inside.

Glaring at me was a face of such beauty that I gasped. The fur was short, smooth, and the rich golden-brown of wild honey. The pointed ears were flattened close to the skull, and the upper lip was drawn back in a series of fine ripples from milk-white teeth and pink gums. But it was the eyes I noticed more than anything else: large, and set at a slight slant in the golden face, they stared up at me with a look of such cold fury that I was thankful the animal's feet were tied. They were

green, the green of leaves under ice, and they glittered like
mica in the evening sun. For a second we stared at each other,
then the Golden Cat drew back her lips even farther away
from her gums, opened her mouth and gave another of those
loud and frightening cries. Hastily I tied the sack up again, for
I did not know if her bonds were really strong or not, and,
judging by her eyes, she would not deal with me very kindly
if she got free.

'You like?' asked the Fon.

'Wah! I like dis beef *too much*,' I replied.

We carried the precious sack up on to the veranda, and I
hastily turned a specimen out of the largest and strongest cage
I had. Then we emptied the Golden Cat gently out of the sack
and rolled her inside, shutting and bolting the door. She lay
on her side, hissing and snarling, but unable to move, for her
front and back legs were neatly tied together with strong
raffia-like cord. By fixing a knife to the end of a stick I managed to saw through these cords, and as they fell away she got
to her feet in one smooth movement, leapt at the bars, stuck
a fat golden paw through, and took a swipe at my face. I drew
back only just in time.

'Aha!' said the Fon, chuckling, 'dis beef get angry too much.'

''E fit chop man time no dere,' said the hunter.

''E get power,' agreed the Fon, nodding, ''e get plenty
power for 'e foot. You go watch um, my friend, less 'e go
wound you.'

I sent down to the kitchen for a small chicken, and this,
freshly killed and warm, I dangled near the bars of the cage. A
golden paw again shot out between the bars, white claws
buried themselves in the fowl and it was jerked up against the
bars. Leaning forward, the cat got a grip on the neck of the
bird, and with one quick heave the entire fowl vanished into
the cage, and clouds of feathers started to pour out from
between the bars as the Golden Cat began to feed. Reverently
I covered the front of the cage with a sack and we left her in
peace to enjoy her meal.

'How you done catch dis beef?' I asked the hunter. He
gave a grin and wiggled his toes with embarrassment.

'You no de hear?' asked the Fon, 'you no get mouth? Speak now!'

'Masa,' began the man, scratching his stomach, 'de Fon done tell me Masa want dis kind of beef too much, an' so three days I done go for bush, I look um. I done walka, walka, I done tire too much, but I never see dis beef. Yesterday, for evening time, dis bushcat 'e done come softly for my farm, an' 'e done chop three chicken. Dis morning I see 'e foot for de mud, an' I done follow for bush. Far too much I done follow um, Masa, an' den, for some big hill, I done see um.'

The Fon shifted in his chair and fixed the man with a glittering eye.

'You speak true?' he asked sternly.

'Yes, Masa,' protested the hunter, 'I speak true.'

'Good,' said the Fon.

'I done see dis bushcat,' the man went on; ''e done walka for dis big hill. Den 'e done go for some place dere be rock too much. 'E done go for hole in de ground. I look dis hole, but man no fit pass, 'e tight too much. I done go back for my house an' I done bring fine dog and catchnet, den I go back for dis place. I done put catchnet for de hole, an' den I done make small fire an' put smoke for de hole.'

He paused and hopped on one leg, clicking his fingers.

'Wah! Dat beef fierce too much! When 'e done smell de smoke 'e de hollar an' 'e de hollar, time no dere. My dog dey de fear an' dey all done run. I de fear bushcat go catch me an' I done run also. Small time I hear de beef 'e hollar an' hollar, an' so I done go softly softly for look um. Wah! Masa, dat beef 'e run run for inside catchnet, an' de catchnet done hold um fine. When I see um for catchnet I no get fear again, an' so I done go an' tie 'e foot with rope, an' I done bring um one time for Masa.'

The man ended his story and stood watching us anxiously, twisting his short spear in both hands.

'My friend,' I told him, 'I tink you be fine hunter man, an' I go pay you good money for dis beef.'

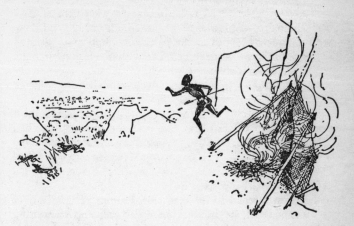

'Na so, na so,' agreed the Fon, waving a lordly hand, 'dis man done make fine hunting for you.'

I paid him a handsome sum of money, and made him a present of several packets of cigarettes, and he went off grinning and ejaculating, 'Tank you, Masa, tank you,' all the way down the steps and along the road until he was out of earshot. Then I turned to the Fon, who was sitting back watching me with a smug expression on his face.

'My friend, I tank you too much for dis ting you done do,' I said.

The Fon waved his hands deprecatingly.

'No, no, my friend, na small ting dis. It no be good ting if you go leave Bafut and you never get all de beef you want. I sorry too much you do go leave. But, when you look dis fine beef you go tink of Bafut, no be so?'

'Na true,' I said, 'and now, my friend, you go drink with me?'

'Foine, foine,' said the Fon.

As if to compensate for the dreariness of the early part of the day, the sunset was one of the finest I have ever seen. The sun sank down behind a grid of pale, elongated clouds, and as it sank, the clouds turned from white to pearly pink, and then flushed to crimson edged with gold. The sky itself was washed with the palest of blues and greens, smudged here and there with a touch of gold, with pale, trembling stars gaining strength as the world darkened. Presently the moon came up, blood-red at first, changing to yellow and then silver as she rose, turning the world a frosty silver, with shadows as black as charcoal.

The Fon and I sat drinking in the misty moonlight until it was late. Then he turned to me, pointing towards his villa.

'I tink sometime you like to dance,' he said, 'so I done tell um to make musica. You like we go dance before you leave, eh?'

'Yes, I like to dance,' I said.

The Fon lurched to his feet, and, leaning perilously over the veranda rail, he shouted an order to someone waiting below. In a short time a cluster of lights moved across the great courtyard, and the Fon's all-female band assembled in the road below and started to play. Soon they were joined by numerous others, including most of the council members. The Fon listened to the music for a bit, waving his hands and smiling, and then he got up and held out his hand to me.

'Come!' he said, 'we go dance, eh?'

'Foine, foine!' I mimicked him, and he crowed with glee.

We made our way across the moon-misty veranda to the head of the steps; the Fon draped a long arm over my shoulders, partly out of affection and partly for support, and we started to descend. Half-way down, my companion stopped to execute a short dance to the music. His foot got tangled up in his impressive robes, and, but for his firm grip round my neck he would have rolled down the steps into the road. As it was, we struggled there for a moment, swaying violently, as we tried to regain our balance; the crowd of wives, offspring, and councillors gave a great gasp of horror and consternation at the sight of their lord in such peril, and the band stopped playing.

'Musica, musica!' roared the Fon, as we reeled together on the steps; 'why you done stop, eh?'

The band started up again, we regained our equilibrium and

walked down the rest of the way without mishap. The Fon was in fine fettle, and he insisted on holding my hand and dancing across the courtyard, splashing through the puddles, while the band trotted behind, playing a trifle short-windedly. When we reached the dancing-hut he sat down on his throne for a rest, while his court took the floor. Presently, when there was a slight lull in the dancing, I asked the Fon if he would call the band over, so that I could examine the instruments more closely. They trooped over and stood in front of the dais on which we sat, while I tried each instrument in turn and was shown the correct way of playing it. To everyone's surprise, including my own, I succeeded in playing the first few bars of 'The Campbells are Coming' on a bamboo flute. The Fon was so delighted with this that he made me repeat it several times while he accompanied me on a big drum, and one of the council members on the strange foghorn-like instrument. The effect was not altogether musical, but we rendered it with great verve and feeling. Then we had to repeat it all over again, so that the Fon could hear how it sounded with a full band accompaniment. Actually, it sounded rather good, as most of my flat notes were drowned by the drums.

When we had exhausted the musical possibilities of the tune, the Fon sent for another bottle, and we settled down to watch the dancers. The inactivity soon told on my companion, and after an hour or so he started to shift on his throne and to scowl at the band. He filled up our glasses, and then leant back and glared at the dancers.

'Dis dance no be good,' he confided at last.

'Na fine,' I said; 'why you no like?'

''E slow too much,' he pointed out, and then he leant over and smiled at me disarmingly, 'You like we go dance your special dance?'

'Special dance?' I queried, slightly fuddled; 'what dance?'

'One, two, three, keek; one, two, three, keek,' yodelled the Fon.

'Ah, dat dance you de talk. Yes, we go dance um if you like.'

'I like too much,' said the Fon firmly.

He led the way on to the dance-floor, and clutched my waist in a firm grip, while everyone else, all chattering and grinning with delight, joined on behind. In order to add a little variety to the affair I borrowed a flute, and piped noisily and inaccurately on it as I led them on a wild dance round the dance hall and out among the huts of the Fon's wives. The night was warm, and half an hour of this exercise made me stream with sweat and gasp for breath. We stopped for a rest and some liquid refreshment. It was obvious, however, that my Conga had got into the Fon's blood. He sat on his throne, his eyes gleaming, feet tapping, humming reminiscently to himself, and obviously waiting with ill-concealed impatience until I had recovered my breath before suggesting that we repeat the whole performance. I decided that I would have to head him off in some way, for I found the Conga too enervating for such a close night, and I had barked my shin quite painfully on a door-post during our last round. I cast around in my mind for another dance I could teach him which would be less strenuous to perform, and yet whose tune could be easily mastered by the band. I made my choice, and then called once more for a flute, and practised on it for a few minutes. Then I turned to the Fon, who had been watching me with great interest.

'If you go tell de band 'e go learn dis special music I go teach you other European dance,' I said.

'Ah! Foine, foine,' he said, his eyes gleaming, and he turned and roared the band to silence, and then marshalled them round the dais while I played the tune to them. In a surprisingly short time they had picked it up, and were even adding little variations of their own. The Fon stamped his feet delightedly.

'Na fine music dis,' he said; 'now you go show me dis dance, eh?'

I looked round and singled out a young damsel, who I had noticed, seemed exceptionally bright, and, clasping her as closely as propriety would permit (for her clothing was non-existent), I set off across the dance-floor in a dashing polka. My partner after only a momentary hesitation picked up the step perfectly, and we bobbed and hopped round in great style. To show his appreciation of this new dance, the Fon started to clap, and immediately the rest of the court followed suit; it started off as normal, ragged applause; but, being Africans, our audience kept clapping and worked it into the rhythm of the dance. The girl and I circled round the large floor five times, and then we were forced to stop for a rest. When I reached the dais, the Fon held out a brimming glass of whisky for me and clapped me on the back as I sat down.

'Na foine dance!' he said.

I nodded and gulped down my drink. As soon as I had put my glass down, the Fon seized me by the hand and pulled me on to the floor again.

'Come,' he said persuasively, 'you go show me dis dance.'

Clasped in each other's arms, we polkaed round the room, but it was not a great success, chiefly because my partner's robes became entangled with my feet and jerked us both to a halt. We would then have to stand patiently while a crowd of council members unwound us, after which away we would go again: one, two, three, hop, only to end up in the opposite corner entwined together like a couple of maypoles.

Eventually I glanced at my watch and discovered to my dismay that it was three o'clock. Reluctantly I had to take my leave of the Fon and retire to bed. He and the court followed me out into the great courtyard, and there I left them. As I climbed up the steps to the villa I looked back at them. In among the twinkling hurricane lanterns they were all dancing the polka. In the centre of them the Fon was jigging and hopping by himself, waving one long arm and shouting 'Good night, my friend, good night!' I waved back, and then went and crawled thankfully into my bed.

By eight-thirty the next morning the lorry had arrived and the collection had been stacked on to it. An incredible number of Bafutians had come to say good-bye and to see me off; they had been arriving since early that morning, and now lined the roadside, chattering together, waiting for me to depart. The last load was hoisted on to the lorry, and the sound of drums, flutes, and rattles heralded the arrival of the Fon to take his leave of me. He was dressed as I had seen him on the day of my arrival, in a plain white robe and a wine-red skull-cap. He was accompanied by his retinue of highly-coloured councillors. He strode up and embraced me, and then, holding me by the hand, addressed the assembled Bafutians in a few rapid sentences. When he stopped, the crowd broke into loud 'arrr's' and started to clap rhythmically. The Fon turned to me and raised his voice.

'My people 'e sorry too much you go leave Bafut. All dis people dey go remember you, and you no go forget Bafut, eh?'

'I never go forget Bafut,' I said truthfully, making myself heard with difficulty above the loud and steady clapping of those hundreds of black hands.

'Good,' he said with satisfaction; then he clasped my hand firmly in his and wrung it. 'My friend always I go get you for my eye. I no go forget dis happy time we done get. By God power you go reach your own country safe. Walka good, my friend, walka good.'

As the lorry started off down the road the clapping got faster and faster, until it sounded like rain on a tin roof. We jolted our way slowly along until we reached the corner; looking back I saw the road lined with naked black humanity, their hands fluttering as they clapped, and at the end of this avenue of moving hands and flashing teeth stood a tall figure in dazzling white. It raised a long arm, and a huge hand waved a last farewell as the lorry rounded the corner and started up the red earth road that wound over the golden, glittering hills.

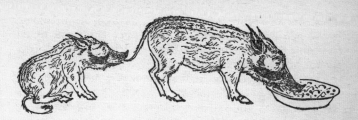

CHAPTER TEN

Zoo under Canvas

ONE of the most frustrating things for the collector is that he can rarely get to know any of his animals until towards the end of a trip. During the first four months or so they are just specimens to him, for he has not the time to observe them closely enough for them to assume characters of their own. He sees that they are adequately housed, feeds and cleans them; but beyond that he cannot go, for all his spare time is spent in trying to add to his menagerie. Towards the end of a trip, however, his collection has grown to such proportions that he cannot wander far afield, for he has too much to do. Then is the time when he has to rely entirely on the native hunters to bring in new specimens, and he, being confined to camp all day, has the opportunity of getting to know the creatures he has already assembled. Our collection had reached such a point when I returned from Bafut. Not only had we the grassland animals, but during my stay in the mountains Smith had been steadily increasing the collection with the local forest fauna. Under the great canvas roof of our marquee we had a large and varied enough collection of creatures to start a small zoo.

So, on my return to our hot and humid base camp on the banks of the Cross River, I began to appreciate some of my grassland captures for the first time. For example, take the case of the hyrax. Until I got them down to base camp I had considered them to be rather dull creatures, whose only claim to fame was their relatives. At first glance one would be pardoned for mistaking a hyrax for an ordinary member of the great group of rodents, and as you watched them nibbling away at leaves or gnawing at some juicy bark, you would probably hazard a guess that they were related to the rabbits. In this you would be quite wrong, for a hyrax is an ungulate, an order which includes cattle, deer, swine, and horses; and the nearest relative to the hyrax is not the rabbit but the elephant, of all unlikely things. In the bone formation of the feet, and in other anatomical details, the hyrax is classified as coming closer to the elephant and the rhino than anything else. This is the sort of information that makes people wonder whether zoologists are quite sane, for a hyrax resembles an elephant about as closely as an elephant does a humming-bird. However, the relationship is clearer if one goes into the more complicated details of anatomy and dentition. This, frankly, was all the information I had about the hyrax.

When I reached base camp, the old female hyrax, which had savaged the Beagle's foot, and her two fat babies were transferred from the small cage they had been confined in to a much bigger affair that gave them plenty of space to move about in and had a private bedroom to which to retire if they felt in any way anti-social. In this cage I noticed several things about them which I had not observed before. To begin with, they had what are called 'lavatory habits'; that is to say, they always deposited their dirt in one spot in the cage. Until then I had not realized what a godsend an animal with these habits could be to a hard-working collector. As soon as I had grasped the meaning of the neat little pile of dung I found in the corner of the cage each morning, I set about making the cleaning of the hyrax cage a much simpler operation. I simply provided them with a round, shallow tin as a latrine. To my annoyance, the next morning I found that they had spurned my offer; they had simply pushed the tin out of the way and deposited their dirt in the usual place in the normal fashion. So that night I put the tin in again, but this time I placed a few of their droppings in the bottom. The following day, to my delight, the tin was piled high with dirt, and the floor of the cage was spotless. After that the cleaning of the cage took approximately five minutes: you simply emptied the tin, washed and replaced it in the corner. It became a real pleasure to clean out the hyrax.

As a contrast in habits there were the Pouched Rats: these rodents, each as large as a small kitten, lived in the cage next door to the hyrax family. These belonged to that irritating group of beasts that won't – or can't – evacuate their bowels unless it is done into water, and preferably running water. In the wild state they would probably use a stream for this purpose, and the current would carry the dirt away to fertilize some plant farther downstream. In a cage, however, I could not provide the Pouched Rats with a stream, so they used the next best thing, which was their water-pot. There is nothing quite so frustrating as putting a nice clean water-pot, brimming with clear liquid, into a cage, and, on looking at it five minutes later, finding that it resembles a pot full of liquid manure. It was very worrying, for in the heat the animals needed a constant supply of fresh drinking-water, and yet here were the rats dirtying their water before drinking it. After many futile attempts to get them to abandon this habit, I used to supply them with a large pot of water as a lavatory, and plenty of juicy fruit to eat, in the hope that this would quench their thirst.

But to return to the hyrax: in Bafut I had decided that they were dull, unfriendly animals who spent their whole lives sitting on their haunches chewing leaves with a glazed look in their eyes. At base camp I discovered that I was quite mistaken, for a hyrax can be as lively as a lamb when it puts its mind to it. In the evening, when their cage was flooded with sunlight, the old female would lie there looking as imposing as a Trafalgar Square lion, munching methodically at a bunch of tender spinach, or a cluster of cassava leaves, while her babies played with each other. These were wild and exhilarating romps they used to have: they would chase one another round and round the cage, sometimes astonishing me by running straight up the smooth wooden back of the cage until they reached the roof before dropping off on to the floor. When they tired of these Wall-of-Death stunts they would use their mother's portly and recumbent body as a castle. One would climb up on to her back, while the other would attack and try to knock him off.

Occasionally they would both be on their mother's back together, locked in mortal combat, while their parent lay there unmoved, chewing steadily, a trance-like look on her face. These games were delightful to watch, but there was one annoying thing about them, and this was that the babies would sometimes carry on far into the night, especially if there was a moon. It is extremely difficult to get to sleep when a pair of baby hyrax are dashing about their cage, producing a noise like a couple of stallions fighting in a loose-box. Sitting up in bed and shouting 'SHUT UP' in fearsome tones had the effect of stopping them for about half an hour; if you had not drifted into sleep by then, you would be brought back to life once again by the thumping of wood, twanging of wire, and the melodious crash of food-pots being kicked over. The hyrax were certainly anything but dull.

Another creature that started to blossom into his true colours when we arrived at base camp was the Black-eared Squirrel, the beast that had created such havoc on the steps of the villa in Bafut. This episode of the steps was, if I had only known it at the time, but a slight indication of what he could do when he put his mind to it, for his one delight in life seemed to consist in escaping and being chased by a crowd of people. He was, as I have already mentioned, quite a baby, and within a very short time after his arrival he had become extraordinarily tame and would allow me to pick him up and place him on my shoulder, where he would sit up on his hind legs and investigate my ear, in the hope that I had been sensible enough to secrete a palm-nut or some other delicacy there. As long as there were not more than four people about, he would behave with the utmost decorum; a crowd, however, filled him with the unholy desire to be chased. At first I thought that a crowd of people worried and frightened him and that he ran away to try to escape from them. I soon discovered that it was nothing of the sort, for if he found his pursuers lagging behind, he would stop, sit up on his hind legs, and wait for them to catch up. There was a certain humour in the fact that we had christened the little brute Sweeti-pie (because of his docility and nice nature) before we discovered his vice. The first race organized by Sweeti-pie took place three days after we had arrived at the marquee.

Our water supply for the camp was kept in two great petrol drums which stood near the kitchen. These were filled every day by the convicts from the local prison. They were a cheerful group of men, clad in spotless white smocks and shorts, who toiled up the hill to camp every morning carrying brimming kerosene tins of water on their shaven heads. Behind them would walk a warder in an i .pressive fawn uniform, his brass buttons flashing in the sun, swinging a short truncheon with a capable air. The convicts, whose crimes ranged from petty theft to manslaughter, went about their tedious task with great good humour, and when you greeted them they would all beam with pleasure. Once a week I distributed a couple of packets of cigarettes among them, and they would be allowed by their warder (who was having a glass of beer with me) to wander round the camp and look at our collection of animals. They thoroughly enjoyed this break in routine, and they would cluster round the monkeys and double up with laughter at their antics, or else peer into the snake-box and give themselves thrills.

On this particular morning when the convicts arrived I was on my way to feed Sweeti-pie. The convicts filed past me, their faces gleaming with sweat, grinning amicably, and greeting me with, 'Morning, Masa. We done come ... we done bring water for Masa ... Iseeya, Masa ...', and so on. The warder gave me a frightfully military salute, and then grinned like a small boy. While they were emptying the contents of their tins into the petrol drums, I got Sweeti-pie out of his cage, sat him on the palm of my hand, and gave him a lump of sugar to eat. He seized the sugar in his mouth and then, glancing round, he saw the group of convicts near the kitchen, exchanging gossip and saucy badinage with the staff. Having made sure that there were enough people there to give him a good run for his money, he took a firmer grip on his sugar, leapt lightly off my hand, and galloped off across the camp clearing, his tail streaming out behind him like a flame in a draught. I set off in pursuit, but before I had gone more than a few paces

Sweeti-pie had gained the thick bushes at the edge of the clearing and dived out of sight. Thinking that it would be the last I should see of him, I uttered such a wail of anguish that everyone dropped what they were doing and ran towards me.

'Dat beef done run,' I yelled to the convicts, 'I go pay five shillings to man who catch um.'

The results of my offer were quite startling: the convicts dropped their kerosene tins and rushed off into the bushes, closely followed by their warder, who discarded both truncheon and hat in case they hampered his movements. The entire staff also joined in the hunt, and the whole crowd of them went crashing through the bushes and short undergrowth in search of Sweeti-pie. They combed the area thoroughly without finding any signs of the animal, and then it was discovered that the little brute had been sitting in the branches of a small bush, watching the search sweep to and fro around him, quietly finishing off his sugar-lump. When he saw that he was spotted, he leapt to the ground, ran through the camp clearing and out on to the path leading away over the hill, hotly pursued by a panting mob consisting of warder, convicts, and staff. They all disappeared from view over the skyline and peace descended on the camp. But not for long, for in a few minutes Sweeti-pie appeared again over the brow of the hill, galloped down into camp, shot through the marquee, and scrambled into his cage, where he innocently started to eat a piece of sugar-cane. Half an hour later the warder, the convicts, and the staff straggled back to camp, all hot and perspiring, to report that the animal had escaped them and was now doubtless deep in the bush. When I showed them Sweeti-pie (who had now finished his meal and was quietly sleeping) and told them how he had returned, they gaped at me for a minute in amazement. And then, being Africans, the humour of the situation struck them and they reeled around the camp yelling with laughter, slapping their thighs, the tears streaming down their faces. The warder was so overcome that he collapsed on the neck of one of the convicts and sobbed with mirth.

Every day after that the warder and the convicts would bring some offering to the beef that had made them run so fast

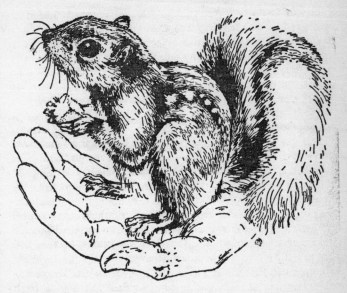

and 'fooled them too much': sometimes it was a bit of sugar-cane, or a handful of groundnuts, sometimes a bit of cassava or a piece of bread. Whatever it was, Sweeti-pie would sit up at the wire and receive the offering with squeaks of pleasure, while the convicts would gather round and relate to each other, or to any new member of their group, the story of how they had chased the squirrel. Then there would be much laughter, and Sweeti-pie would be praised for his skilful evasive tactics. This was only the first of many occasions when Sweeti-pie caused havoc in the camp.

Of the many different creatures that were brought to us while we were at base camp, about a fifth were babies, and, although they were charming little things for the most part, they caused a great deal of extra work for us, for very young animals require just as much care and attention as a human baby. All these young creatures endeared themselves to us, but one of the most charming and, at the same time, irritating trios of beasts we acquired were three little fellows that we called the Bandits. These animals were Kusimanses, a kind of mongoose which is fairly common in the forest. When adult, they are about the size of a large guinea-pig, clad in thick, coarse chocolate fur, a bushy tail, and a long pointed face with a rubbery pink nose and circular protuberant boot-button eyes. The Bandits, when they arrived, were about the size of small rats and had only just got their eyes open. Their fur was a bright gingery colour, and it stuck up in tufts and sprigs all over their bodies, making them look rather like hedgehogs. Their noses were the most prominent part of their anatomy, long and bright pink, and so flexible that they could be whiffled from side to side like a miniature elephant's trunk. At first they had to be fed on milk mixed with calcium and cod-liver oil, and this was no easy task; they drank more milk than any other baby animal I have ever met, and the whole business was made more difficult because they were far too small to suck it out of the feeding-bottle I used for the others. So they had to be fed by wrapping a lump of cotton wool round a stick, dipping it in the milk and then letting them suck it. This work-ed admirably at first, but as soon as their sharp little teeth began to appear through the gums, they started to be trouble-some. They were so greedy that they would take hold of the cotton wool and hang on to it like bulldogs, refusing to let go and allow me to dip it into the milk again. On many occasions they would grip so hard that the cotton wool would come off the end of the stick, and then they would try to swallow it; only by sticking my finger down their throats and capturing the cotton wool as it was disappearing could I save them from being choked to death. Sticking a finger down their throats always made them sick, and, of course, as soon as they had been sick they would feel hungry again, so the whole perform-ance would have to be repeated. Anyone who prides himself on his patience should try hand-rearing some baby Kusimanses.

When their teeth had come through and they had learnt to walk really well they became most inquisitive and were always trying to push their pink noses into someone else's business. They lived in what we called the nursery – a collection of baskets that housed all the baby animals – and were placed between our two beds, where they were within easy reach for any bottle feeds that had to be given at night. The top of the basket which the Bandits inhabited was not too secure, and it was not long before they learnt how to push it off; then they would scramble out and go on a tour of inspection round the camp. This was extremely worrying, for the Bandits seemed to be completely lacking in fear and would stick their noses into monkey cages or snake-boxes with equal freedom. Their lives were devoted to a search for food, and everything they came across they would bite in the hope that it would turn out to be tasty. At that time we had a fully grown female Colobus monkey, a creature which possessed a wonderfully long, thick coat of silky black and white hair, and a long, plume-like tail, also black and white, of which she seemed very proud, for she was always most particular about keeping it clean and glossy. One day the Bandits escaped from the nursery and wandered round by the monkey cages to see what they could pick up. The Colobus was reclining on the bottom of her cage having a sun bath, and her long and beautiful tail was sticking out between the bars and lying on the ground. One of the Bandits discovered this curious object and, since it did not appear to belong to anyone, he rushed at it and sank his sharp little teeth into it to see whether it was edible. The other two, seeing what he had found, immediately joined him and laid hold of the tail as well. The unfortunate monkey, screaming loudly with rage and fright, scrambled up to the top of her cage, but this did not shake off the Bandits; they clung on like a vice, and the higher the Colobus climbed in her cage, the higher her tail lifted the Bandits off the ground. When I arrived on the scene they were suspended about a foot in the air, and were hanging there, revolving slowly, all growling through clenched teeth. It took me several minutes to induce them to let go, and then they did so only because I blew cigarette smoke into their faces and made them cough.

When the Bandits became old enough to have a special cage of their own, complete with bedroom, feeding them was a job fraught with great difficulty and danger. They grew so excited at meal-times that they would fasten their teeth into

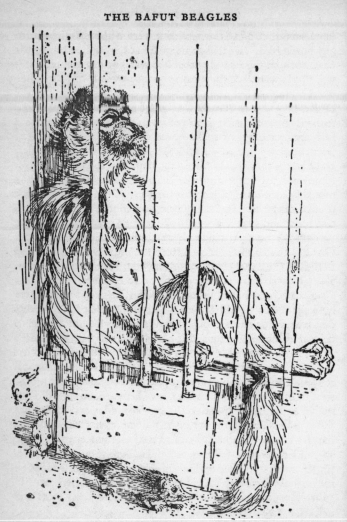

anything that looked even remotely like food, so that you had
to watch your hands. Instead of waiting until the food dish
was put inside their cage, like any sensible animal, they would
leap through the door to meet it, knock the dish out of your

hand, and then fall to the ground in a tangled heap, all screaming loudly with frustrated rage. Eventually I became rather
tired of having the Bandits shoot out like ginger rockets every
time I went to feed them, so I evolved a plan. Two of us
would approach the cage at meal-times, and the Bandits would
hurl themselves at the bar, screaming loudly, their eyes pop-
ping with emotion. Then one of us would rattle the bedroom
door, and they, thinking that the food was being put in there,
would throw themselves into the sleeping quarters, fighting
and scrambling to get there first. While they were thus engaged you had exactly two seconds' grace before they found
out the deception: during that time you had to open the cage
door, put the food inside and withdraw your hand and lock
the door again. If you were not quick, or made some slight
noise to attract their attention, the Bandits would tumble out
of the bedroom, screeching and chittering, upset the plate, and
bite indiscriminately at the food and your hand. It was all very
trying.

About this time we had another pair of babies brought to us,
who proved to be full of charm and personality. They were a
pair of baby Red River Hogs and, as with the Kusimanses, they
looked totally unlike the adult. A fully grown Red River Hog
is probably the most attractive member of the pig family, and
certainly the most highly coloured. They have bright rusty-
orange fur, with deeper, almost chocolate markings round the
snout. Their large ears end in two extraordinary pencil-like
tufts of pure white hair, and a mane of this white hair runs
along their backs. The two babies were, like all young pigs,
striped: the ground colour was a deep brown, almost black,
and from snout to tail they were banded with wide lines of
bright mustard-yellow fur, a colour scheme that had the effect
of making them look more like fat wasps than baby pigs.

The little male was the first to arrive, sitting forlornly in
a basket carried on the head of a brawny hunter. He was
obviously in need of a good feed of warm milk, and as soon as
I had paid for him I prepared a bottle and then lifted him out
on to my knee. He was about the size of a pekinese, and had
very sharp little hooves and tusks, as I soon found out. He had

never seen a feeding-bottle and treated it with the gravest suspicion from the start. When I lifted him on to my knee and tried to get the teat into his mouth, he kicked and squealed, ripping my trousers with his hooves and trying to bite with his tiny tusks. At the end of five minutes we both looked as though we had bathed in milk, but not a drop of it had gone down his throat. In the end I had to hold him firmly between my knees, wedge his mouth open with one hand while squirting milk in with the other. As soon as the first few drops trickled down his throat he stopped struggling and screaming, and within a few minutes he was sucking away at the bottle as hard as he could go. After this he was no more trouble, and within two days had lost all his fear of me, and would come running to the bars of his pen when I appeared, squeaking and grunting with delight, rolling over on to his back to have his bulging stomach scratched.

The female piglet arrived a week later, and she was brought in protesting so loudly that we could hear her long before she and the hunter came in sight. She was almost twice the size of the male, so I decided that they must have separate cages to start with, as I was afraid that she might hurt him. But when I put her in the pen next door to him, their obvious delight at seeing each other, and the way they rushed to the intervening bars, squeaking and rubbing noses, made me decide that they should share a cage straight away. When I put them together the tiny male ran forward, sniffing loudly, and butted the female gently in the ribs; she snorted and skipped away across the cage. He chased her, and together they ran round and round the cage, twisting and turning and doubling back with astonishing agility for such portly beasts. When they had worked off their high spirits, they burrowed deep into the pile of dry banana leaves I had provided for them and fell asleep, snoring like a beehive on a summer night.

The female, being so much older, very soon learnt to supplement her bottle-feed with a dish of chopped fruit and vegetables. After giving both of them their bottle I would put a broad, shallow pan full of this mixture into the cage, and she would spend the morning standing there with her nose buried in it, making slushy, squelching piggy noises and sighing dreamily at intervals. The little male could not understand this, and he used to become very incensed at being ignored; he would go and prod her with his snout, or nibble at her legs, until she would suddenly turn on him with squeals of rage and drive him away. He tried several times to see what it was in the dish that was attracting her, but could not discover anything very exciting about a lot of chopped fruit, so he would wander off moodily and sit in a corner by himself until she had finished. One day, however, he decided that he, too, could get an extra meal, by the simple expedient of sucking the female's long tail. He became convinced that if he sucked it long enough and hard enough he would get milk from it. So she used to stand there with her nose buried in the dish of food, while behind her stood the male with her tail held hopefully in his mouth. This did not seem to worry her unduly, but he sucked so enthusiastically that her tail became quite bald, and in order to let the hair grow again I had to keep them in separate cages, only allowing them to be with one another for a game twice a day.

Life in the marquee with half a hundred animals to look after was anything but dull. We were surrounded on all sides by animals of all shapes, sizes, and kinds, from tree-frogs to owls, and from pythons to monkeys. At all hours of the day and night a steady mutter of strange noises filled the air – noises that ranged from the maniacal screams and giggles of the chimpanzees to the steady rasping sound of a Pouched Rat who was convinced that, by sticking to it in spite of all opposition, he could gnaw his way through a metal feeding-pot. At any time of the day you could find something to do, or something new to note or observe. The following extracts from a week's entries in my diary give some indication of the wealth of small but exciting or interesting incidents that were worth noting:

The young female Stanger's Squirrel's eyes have now changed from that beautiful shade of sky blue to steel grey; when you disturb her at night she makes a noise like a clockwork train when it is lifted off the rails . . . one of the Palm Vipers has given birth to eleven young: about five inches long, ground colour pale slate grey with cross bands of dark ash grey, making wonderful contrast to vivid green and white mother; they all struck viciously at a stick when only a couple of hours old ... large green tree frogs make a noise like a clock slowly ticking, just before rain, but will stop if you go near their cage, and won't perform again until next cloudburst ... discovered that the galagos like the flowers of a species of marigold that grows around here; they hold flower head in one hand and pluck off petals with the other, cramming them into their mouths; then they play with the remains as though it were a shuttlecock, looking quite ridiculous, with their great eyes staring ...

Feeding notes: Golden Cat adores brain and liver chopped up and mixed with raw egg – exotic tastes some of these beasts have! Pangolins [Scaly Anteaters] won't eat their egg and milk mixture if it's sweetened, but simply overturn dish – extremely annoying! Fruit Bats prefer their bananas to be given with the skins on; they eat the whole lot, and the skin seems to prevent their bowels from becoming too loose. Over-ripe fruit causes havoc among the monkey bowels (especially chimps – messy!), yet the bats will eat and enjoy without ill-effects fruit that is fermenting, providing there is roughage with it. Too much goat meat causes rupture of the anus in the Marsh Mongooses, for some peculiar reason; warm cod-liver oil and *very gentle* pressure will get it back into place; animal will become very exhausted and then one drop whisky in tablespoon of water helps them.

These were the little things that made up life in the base camp, but they were of absorbing interest to us, and the days seemed so full of colour and incident that they sped past unnoticed. So it is not surprising that I was rather terse with a pleasant but stupid young man who said, after being shown round the collection, 'Don't you ever go out and have a pot at a monkey or something? Should have thought you would have died of boredom, stuck down here all day with this lot.'

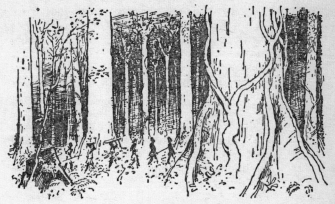

CHAPTER ELEVEN

The Forest of Flying Mice

WHEN I returned from the mountains to our Cross River base
camp there was only one gap of importance in our collection.
The gap was noticeable to me, for it was caused by the absence
of a tiny animal which I wanted to catch more than practically
any other creature in the Cameroons. The English name for
this beast is the Pigmy Scaly-tail, while zoologists, in their
usual flippant and familiar manner, call it *Idiurus kivuensis*.
When in England I had pored over drawings and museum
skins of the beast, and since our arrival in Africa I had talked
about it incessantly, until even the staff knew that *Idiurus kivuensis* was the name of a beef that I prized beyond all measure.

I knew that *Idiurus* was a strictly nocturnal animal; it was,
moreover, only the size of a small mouse, which made it unlikely that any of the hunters would know it. I was right, for
they did not recognize the drawing I had. From the small
amount of literature dealing with the species I had managed to
glean the fact that they lived in colonies in hollow trees, pre-
ferring the less accessible portions of the forest. I explained
this to the hunters, in the faint hope that it would spur them

on to search for specimens, but it was no use; the African will not hunt for an animal he has never seen, for he considers it likely that it may not exist – to hunt for it would be a waste of time. I had had precisely the same trouble over the Hairy Frogs, so I realized that my tales of small small rats that flew like birds from tree to tree were doomed from the start. One thing was very clear: if I wanted *Idiurus* I would have to go out and hunt for it myself, and I should have to do so quickly, for our time was short. I decided to make the village of Eshobi my headquarters for the *Idiurus* hunt; it was a day's march from base camp, in the depths of the forest, and I knew the inhabitants well, for I had stayed there on a previous visit to the Cameroons. Hunting for a creature the size of a mouse in the deep rain-forest that stretches for several hundred miles in all directions may sound like an improved version of the needle-in-the-haystack routine but it is this sort of thing that makes collecting so interesting. My chances of success were one in a thousand, but I set off cheerfully into the forest.

The Eshobi road can only be appreciated by someone with a saint-like predilection for mortifying the flesh. Most of it resembles an old dried watercourse, though it follows a route that no self-respecting river would take. It runs in a series of erratic zig-zags through the trees, occasionally tumbling down a steep slope into a valley, crossing a small stream and climbing up the opposite side. On the downward slope the rocks and stones which made up its surface were always loose, so that on occasions your descent was quicker than you anticipated. As the road started to climb up the opposite side of the valley, however, you would find that the rocks had increased considerably in size and were placed like a series of steps. This was a snare and a delusion, for each rock had been so cunningly placed that it was quite impossible to step from it to the next one. They were all thickly covered with a cloak of green moss, wild begonias, and ferns, so you could not tell, before jumping, exactly what shape your landing ground was going to be.

The track went on like this for some three miles, then we toiled up from the bottom of a deep valley and found that the forest floor was level and the path almost as smooth as a motor road. It wound and twisted its way through the giant trees, and here and there along its length there was a rent in the foliage above, which let through a shaft of sunlight. In these patches of sun, warming themselves after the night's dew, sat a host of butterflies. They rose and flew round us as we walked, dipping and fluttering and wheeling in a sun-drunken condition. There were tiny white ones like fragile chips of snow, great clumsy ones whose wings shone like burnished copper, and others decked out in blacks, greens, reds, and yellows. Once we had passed, they settled again on the sunlit path and sat there gaily, occasionally opening and closing their wings. This ballet of butterflies was always to be seen on the Eshobi path, and is moreover the only life you are likely to see, for the deep forest does not teem with dangerous game, as some books would have you believe.

We followed this path for about three hours, stopping at times so that the sweating carriers could lower their loads to the ground and have a rest. Presently the path curved, and as we rounded a corner the forest ended and we found ourselves walking up the main and only street of Eshobi. Dogs barked, chickens scuttled and squawked out of our way, and a small toddler rose from the dust where he had been playing and fled into the nearest hut, screaming his lungs out. Suddenly, as if from nowhere, we were surrounded by a milling crowd of humanity: men and boys, women of all ages, all grinning and clapping, pushing forward to shake me by the hand.

'Welcome, Masa, welcome!'

'You done come, Masa!'

'Iseeya, Masa, welcome!'

'Eh ... eahh! Masa, you done come back to Eshobi!'

I was escorted down the village street by this welcoming, chattering mob of humanity as though I were royalty. Someone rushed for a chair and I was seated in state with the entire village standing admiringly around me, beaming and ejaculating 'Welcome' at intervals, now and again clapping their hands, or cracking their knuckles, in an excess of delight.

I was still greeting old friends and inquiring after people's relatives and offspring when my carriers and the cook appeared. Then a long argument arose as to where I should stay, and at last the villagers decided that the only place fit for such a distinguished visitor was their newly built dance-hall. This was a very large, circular hut, the floor of which had been worn to the smoothness of planed wood through the trampling and shuffling of hundreds of feet. The band of drums, flutes, and rattles was hastily removed, the floor was swept, and I was installed.

After I had eaten and drunk, the village gathered round once again to hear what I had come for this time. I explained at great length that I had only come for a short visit, and that I wanted only one kind of creature, and I went on to describe *Idiurus*. I showed them a drawing of the animal, and it was passed from hand to hand, and everyone shook their heads over it and said sorrowfully that they had never seen it. My heart sank. Then I picked out three hunters with whom I had worked before. I told them that they were to go to the forest immediately and to hunt for all the hollow trees they could find, and then to mark them. On the following day they would come and tell me what success they had met with, and guide me to the trees they had found. Then I asked if there was any-one present who could climb trees. A dozen or so hands went up. The volunteers were a very mixed crowd, and I eyed them doubtfully.

'You fit climb stick?' I asked.

'Yes sah, we fit,' came the instant and untruthful chorus.

I pointed to an enormous tree that grew at the edge of the village.

'You fit climb dat big stick?' I inquired.

Immediately the number of volunteers dwindled, until at last only one man still had his hand up.

'You fit climb dat big stick?' I repeated, thinking he had not heard.

'Yes, sah,' he said.

'For true?'

'Yes, sah, I fit climb um. I fit climb stick big pass dat one.'

'All right, then you go come for bush with me tomorrow, you hear.'

'Yes, sah,' said the man, grinning.

'Na what they de call you?'

'Peter, sah.'

'Right, you go come tomorrow for early-early morning time.'

The hunters and the other village inhabitants dispersed, and I unpacked my equipment and made ready for the next day. The entire village returned that evening, silently and cautiously, and watched me having my bath. This they were able to do in comparative comfort, for the walls of the dance-hall had many windows and cracks in them. There must have been some fifty people watching me as I covered myself with soap, and sang lustily, but I did not become aware of the fact for quite some time. It did not worry me, for I am not unduly modest, and as long as my audience (half of which consisted of women) were silent and made no ribald remarks I was content that they should watch. However, Jacob arrived at that moment, and was shocked beyond belief at the disgusting inquisitiveness of the villagers. Seizing a stick, he dashed at them and drove them away in a rushing, screaming mob. He returned panting and full of righteous indignation. Soon afterwards I discovered that he had overlooked two of the crowd, for their earnest black faces were wedged in one of the windows. I called Jacob.

'Jacob,' I said, waving a soapy hand at the window, 'they done come back.'

He examined the faces at the window.

'No, sah,' he said seriously, 'dis one na my friends.'

Apparently I was not to be defiled by being watched by an indiscriminate mass of villagers, but any personal friends of Jacob's were in a different category. It was not until later that I learned that Jacob was something of a business man: after driving away the crowd, he had announced that those who would pay him a penny for the privilege of watching me bath would be allowed to return. He did quite a brisk trade among the smaller members of the village, many of whom had never seen a European, and who wanted to settle various bets among each other as to whether or not I was white all over.

Very early the next morning my hunters and my tree-climber appeared. The hunters, it transpired, had found and marked some thirty hollow trees in different parts of the forest. They were however dispersed over such a wide area that it would prove impossible to visit them all in one day, so I decided that we would visit the farthest ones first, and gradually work back towards the village.

The path we followed was a typical bush path, about eighteen inches wide, that coiled and twisted among the trees like a dying snake. At first it led up an extremely steep hillside, through massive boulders, each topped with a patch of ferns and moss and starred with the flowers of a tiny pink primrose-like plant. Here and there the great lianas coiled down from the trees, and lay across our path in strange shapes, curving and twisting like giant pythons. At the top of this steep incline the path flattened out, and ran across the level forest floor between the giant tree-trunks. The interior of the forest is cool, and the light is dim; it flickers through the dense fret-work of leaves, which gives it a curious underwater quality. The forest is not the tangled mass of undergrowth that you read about: it is composed of the enormous pillar-like trunks of the trees, set well apart, and interspersed with the thin undergrowth, the young saplings and low-growing plants that lurk in the half-light. We travelled onwards, following the faint trail, for some four miles, and then one of the hunters stopped and stuck his cutlass into the trunk of a great tree with a ringing 'chunk'.

'Dis na tree dat get hole for inside, sah,' he proclaimed.

At the base of the trunk was a slit, some two feet wide and three feet high; I bent and stuck my head inside, and then twisted round so that I could look up the tree. But if there was a top opening, it was hidden from me by some bend in the trunk, for no light filtered down from above. I sniffed vigorously, but all I could smell was rotting wood. The base of the tree yielded nothing but a few bat droppings and the dried husks of various insects. It did not look a particularly good tree, but I thought we might as well try smoking it out and see what it contained.

Smoking out a big forest tree, when it is only done occasionally, is a thrilling procedure. During my search for *Idiurus* the thrill rather wore off, but this was because we were forced to smoke so many trees a day, and a great proportion of them proved to have nothing inside. Smoking a tree is quite an art. and requires a certain amount of practice before you can perfect it. First, having found your tree and made sure that it is really hollow all the way up, you have to discover whether there are any exit holes farther up the trunk, and if there are you have to send a man up to cover them with nets. Then you drape a net over the main hole at the base of the tree in such a way that it does not interfere with the smoking, and yet prevents anything from getting away. The important thing is to make sure that this net is secure: there is nothing quite so exasperating as to have it fall down and envelop you in its folds just as the creatures inside the tree are starting to come out.

With all your nets in position you have to deal with the problem of the fire: this, contrary to all proverbial expectations, has to be all smoke and no fire, unless you want your specimens roasted. First, a small pile of dry twigs is laid in the opening, soaked with kerosene and set alight. As soon as it is ablaze you lay a handful of green leaves on top, and keep replenishing them. The burning of these green leaves produces scarcely any flame, but vast quantities of pungent smoke, which is immediately sucked up into the hollow of the tree. Your next problem is to make sure that there is not too *much* smoke; for if you are not careful you can quite easily asphyxiate your specimens before they can rush out of the tree. The idea is to strike that happy medium between roasting and suffocation of your quarry. Once the fire has been lit and piled with green leaves, it generally takes about three minutes (depending on the size of the tree) before the smoke percolates to every part and the animals start to break cover.

We smoked our first tree, and all we got out of it was a large and indignant moth. We took down the nets, put out the fire, and continued on our way. The next tree that the hunters had marked was half a mile away, and when we reached it we went through the same procedure. This time it was slightly more exciting, for, although there were no *Idiurus* in the trunk, there was some life: the first thing to break cover was a small gecko, beautifully banded in chocolate and ash-grey. These little lizards are quite plentiful in the deep forest, and you generally find two or three in any hollow tree you smoke. Following hard on the gecko's tail came three creatures which looked, as they crawled hastily out of the smoke, like large brown sausages with a fringe of undulating legs along each side: they were giant millipedes, large, stupid, and completely harmless beasts that are very common all over the forest. The inside of hollow trees is their favourite abode, for their diet is rotten wood. This, it seemed, was the entire contents of the tree. We took down the nets, put out the fire, and went on. The next tree was completely empty, as were the three that followed it. The seventh tree produced a small colony of bats, all of which flew frantically out of a hole at the top as soon as Peter tried to climb the tree.

This laborious process of setting up the nets, smoking the tree, taking down the nets, and moving on to the next tree was repeated fifteen times that day, and towards evening we were sore and smarting from a thousand cuts and bruises, and our throats were rough from breathing in lungfuls of smoke. We were all in the deepest depths of depression, for not only had we caught no *Idiurus*, but we had caught nothing else of any value either. By the time we reached the last tree that we would have time to smoke before it got dark I was so tired that I really felt I did not care whether there were any *Idiurus* in its trunk or not. I squatted on the ground, smoking a cigarette and watching the hunters as they made the preparations. The tree was smoked and nothing whatsoever appeared from inside. The hunters looked at me.

'Take down the nets; we go back for Eshobi,' I said wearily.

Jacob was busily disentangling the net from the trunk, when he paused and peered at something that lay inside the tree. He bent, picked it up, and came towards me.

'Masa want dis kind of beef?' he inquired diffidently.

I glanced up, and received a considerable shock, for there, dangling from his fingers by its long feathery tail, its eyes closed and its sides heaving, was an *Idiurus*. He deposited the mouse-sized creature in my cupped hands, and I peered at it: it was quite unconscious, apparently almost asphyxiated by the smoke.

'Quick, quick, Jacob!' I yelped, in an agony of fear, 'bring me small box for put um ... No, no, *not that one*, a good one ... Now put small leaf for inside ... *small leaf*, you moron, not half a tree ... There, that's right.' I placed the *Idiurus* reverently inside the box, and took another look at him. He lay there quite limp and unconscious, his chest heaving and his tiny pink paws twitching. He looked to me to be on the verge of death; frantically seizing a huge bunch of leaves I fanned him vigorously. A quarter of an hour of this peculiar form of artificial respiration and, to my delight, he started to recover. His eyes opened in a bleary fashion, he rolled on to his stomach and lay there looking miserable. I fanned him for a while longer, and then carefully closed the lid of the box.

While I had been trying to revive the *Idiurus*, the hunters had been grouped round me in a silent and sorrowful circle; now that they saw the creature regain its faculties, they gave broad grins of delight. We hastily searched the inside of the tree to see if there were any more lying about, but we found nothing. This puzzled me considerably, for *Idiurus* was supposed to live in large colonies. To find a solitary one, therefore, would be unusual. I sincerely hoped that the textbooks were not wrong; to catch some specimens from a colony of animals is infinitely easier than trying to track down and capture individuals. However, I could not stop to worry about it then; I wanted to get the precious creature back to the village and out of the small travelling box he was in. We packed up the nets and set off through the twilit forest as speedily as we could. I carried the box containing *Idiurus* in my cupped hands as delicately as if it contained eggs, and at intervals I would fan the creature through the wire gauze top.

When I was safely back in the village dance-hall, I prepared a larger cage for the precious beast, and then moved him into it. This was not so easy, for he had fully recovered from the smoke by now, and scuttled about with considerable speed. At last, without letting him escape, or getting myself bitten, I succeeded in manoeuvring him into the new cage, and then I placed my strongest light next to it in order to have a good look at him.

He was about the size of a common House Mouse, and very similar to it in general shape. The first thing that caught your attention was his tail: it was very long (almost twice as long as his body), and down each side of it grew a fringe of long, wavy hairs, so the whole tail looked like a bedraggled feather. His head was large, and rather domed, with small, pixie-pointed ears. His eyes were pitch black, small, and rather prominent. His rodent teeth, a pair of great bright orange incisors, protruded from his mouth in a gentle curve, so that from the side it gave him a most extraordinarily supercilious expression. Perhaps the most curious part about him was the 'flying' membrane, which stretched along each side of his body. This was a long, fine flap of skin, which was attached to his ankles, and to a long, slightly curved, cartilaginous shaft that grew out from his arm, just behind the elbow. When at rest, his membrane was curled and rucked along the side of his body like a curtain pelmet; when he launched himself into the air, however, the legs were stretched out straight, and the membrane thus drawn taut, so that it acted like the wings of a glider. Later I was to discover just how skilful *Idiurus* could be in the air with this primitive gliding apparatus.

When I had gone to bed that night and switched off the light, I could hear my new specimen rustling and scuttling round his cage, and I imagined what a feast he was making on the variety of foods I had put in there for him. But when dawn came and I crawled sleepily out of bed to have a look, I discovered that he had not eaten anything. I was not unduly worried by this, for some creatures when newly caught refuse to eat until they have settled down in captivity. The length of time this takes varies not only with the species, but with the individual animal. I felt that some time during the day *Idiurus* would come down from the top of the cage, where he was clinging, and eat his fill.

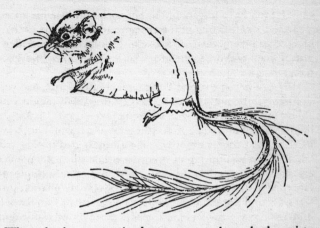

When the hunters arrived we set out through the mist-whitened forest to a fresh series of trees. Refreshed by a night's sleep, and by our capture of an *Idiurus* the day before, we went about the laborious smoking process with a great deal more enthusiasm. But by midday we had investigated ten trees and found nothing. We had by this time reached a section of the forest where the trees were of enormous size, even for the West African forest. They stood well apart from each other, but even so their massive branches interlocked above. The trunks of these trees were, in most cases, at least fifteen feet in diameter. They had great buttress roots – growing out from the base of the trunks like supporting walls of a cathedral, each well over ten feet high where it joined the trunk, and with a space of a good-sized room between each flange. Some of them had wound round them massive, muscular-looking creepers as thick as my body. We made our way through the giant trunks, and came presently to a dip in the level forest floor, a small dell in which stood one of these enormous trees, more or less by itself. At the edge of the dell the hunters paused and pointed.

'Na dis big stick get hole too much, sah,' they said.

We approached the trunk of the tree, and I saw that there was a great arched rent in the wood, between two of the flanges; this hole was about the same size and shape as a small church door. I paused at the entrance to the hole and looked up: the tree-trunk towered above me, shooting up towards the sky smooth and branchless for about two hundred feet. Not a stump, not a branch broke the smooth surface of that column of wood. I began to hope that there would be nothing inside the tree, for I could not see for the life of me how anyone was going to climb up to the top and put nets over the exit holes, if any. I walked into the hollow of the tree as I would walk into a room, and found there was plenty of space; the sunlight filtered gently in through the entrance, and gradually my eyes became accustomed to the dim light. I peered upwards, but a slight bend in the trunk prevented me seeing very far. I tested the sides of the tree and found them composed of rotten wood, soft and spongy. By kicking with my toes I found it was quite easy to make footholds, and I laboriously climbed up the inside of the trunk until I was high enough to crane round the corner. The trunk stretched up as hollow as a factory chimney, and just as big. At the very summit of the tree there was a large exit hole, and through it a shaft of sunlight poured. Then, suddenly, I nearly released my rather precarious hold with excitement, for I saw that the top part of the trunk was literally a moving carpet of *Idiurus*. They slid about on the rotten wood as swiftly and silently as shadows, and when they were still they disappeared completely from sight, so perfectly did they match the background. I slithered to the ground and made my way out into the open. The hunters looked at me expectantly.

'Na beef for inside, Masa?' asked one.

'Yes. Na plenty beef for inside. You go look.'

Chattering excitedly, they pushed and scrambled their way into the inside of the tree; some idea of its size may be gained from the fact that the three hunters, Peter, the tree-climber, and Jacob could all fit comfortably into its spacious interior. I could hear their ejaculations of astonishment as they saw the *Idiurus*, and sharp words being exchanged when someone (I suspected Jacob) trod on somebody else's face in his excitement. I walked slowly round the tree, searching the trunk for any foot or handholds on the bark which would enable Peter to climb to the top, but the bark was as smooth as a billiard ball. As far as I could see, the tree was unclimbable, and I damped the hunters' gaiety by pointing this out to them when they came out of the trunk. While we all sat on the ground and smoked and discussed the matter, Jacob prowled around the dell, scowling ferociously at the trees, and presently he came over to us and said that he thought he had found a way in which Peter could get to the top. We followed him across the dell to its extreme edge, and there he pointed to a tall, thin sapling whose top just reached one of the great branches of the main tree. Jacob suggested that Peter should shin up the sapling, get on to the branch, and then work his way along it until he reached the top of the hollow trunk. Peter examined the sapling suspiciously, and then said he would try. He spat on his hands, seized the trunk of the sapling, and swarmed aloft, using his almost prehensile toes to get extra grip upon the bark. When he reached the half-way mark, however, some seventy feet from the ground, his weight started to bend the sapling over like a bow, and before he had gone much further the trunk was giving ominous creakings. It was obvious that the tree was too slender to support the weight of my corpulent tree-climber, and he was forced to return to earth. Jacob, grinning with excitement, came strutting across to where I stood.

'Masa, I fit climb dat stick,' he said. 'I no be fat man like Peter.'

'Fat!' said Peter indignantly; 'who you de call fat, eh? I no be fat; dat stick no get power for hold man, dat's all.'

'You be fat,' said Jacob scornfully; 'all time you fill your belly with food, an now Masa want you to climb stick you no fit.'

'All right, all right,' I said hastily, 'you go try and climb, Jacob. But take care you no go fall, eh?'

'Yes, sah,' he said, and running to the sapling he flung himself on to the trunk and swarmed up it like a caterpillar.

Now Jacob weighed about half of what Peter weighed, so he was soon clinging to the very tip of the sapling, and the tree was still upright, though it swayed round and round in a gentle curve. Each time it passed the branch of the big tree, Jacob made a wild grab, but each time he missed. Presently he looked down.

'Masa, I no fit catch um,' he called.

'All right, come down,' I shouted back.

He descended rapidly to the ground, and I gave him the end of a long length of strong cord.

'You go tie dis for top, eh? Den, when you ready, we go pull dis small stick so it come for dis big one. Understand?'

'Yes, sah,' said Jacob gleefully, and scuttled up the sapling again.

When he reached the top, he fastened the rope round the sapling and shouted down that he was ready. We laid hold of the rope and pulled lustily; as we backed slowly across the clearing, digging our toes into the soft leaf-mould to gain a grip, the sapling bent slowly over until its tip touched the great branch. Quickly as a squirrel, Jacob had reached out, got a grip on the branch, and hauled himself across. We still held on to the sapling until he had pulled a piece of rope from out of his loin-cloth and tied the top of it to the branch on which he was now lying. When the sapling was tied, we released our hold on the rope gently. Jacob was now standing upright on the branch, holding on to the smaller growth that sprouted from it, and he slowly groped his way along towards the main trunk, walking warily, for the branch he was using as a road was thickly overgrown with orchids, creepers, and tree-ferns, an ideal habitat for a tree-snake. When he reached the place where the branch joined the tree, he squatted astride it, and lowered a long piece of string to us; to the end of this we tied a bundle of nets and some small boxes in which to put any specimens he caught at the top. With these safely tied to his waist he moved round the tree to the hole, which was situated in the crutch where the great branches spread away from the trunk. Squatting down, he spread the net over the hole, arranged the boxes within easy reach, and then grinned down at us mischievously.

'All right, Masa, your hunter man 'e ready now,' he shouted.

'Hunter man!' muttered Peter indignantly; 'dis cook call himself hunter man ... eh ... aehh!'

We collected a mass of dry twigs and green leaves, and laid the fire in the huge chimney-like opening of the tree. We lit it and piled the green leaves on, after draping a net over the arched opening. The fire smouldered sullenly for a few minutes, and then the frail wisp of smoke grew stronger, and soon a great stream of grey smoke was pouring up the hollow shell of the tree. As the smoke rose up the trunk I became aware that there were other holes which we had not spotted, for at various points in the bark, some thirty feet above the ground, frail wisps of smoke started to appear, coiling out and fading into the air.

Jacob, perched precariously, was peering down into the inside of the trunk when the thick column of grey smoke swept up and enveloped him. We could hear him coughing and choking, and could see him moving round gingerly in the smoke, in an effort to find a more suitable spot to sit. It seemed to me, waiting excitedly, that the *Idiurus* took a tremendously long time to be affected by the smoke.

I was just wondering if perhaps they had all been knocked immediately unconscious before they could attempt to escape, when the first one broke cover. It scuttled out of the opening in the base of the tree, tried to launch itself into the air, and became immediately entangled in the nets. One of the hunters rushed forward to disentangle it, but before I could go and help him, the entire colony decided to vacate the tree in a body. Some twenty *Idiurus* appeared at the main opening, and leapt into the net. Up on the top of the tree, now hidden by billows of smoke, I could hear Jacob squeaking with excitement, and occasionally giving a roar of anguish as one of the *Idiurus* bit him. I discovered to my annoyance that there were two or three cracks in the trunk which we had overlooked, some thirty feet above the ground, and through these minute openings the *Idiurus* were swarming out into the open air. They scuttled about the bark, and seemed quite unperturbed by either the strong sunlight or our presence, for some of them came down to within six feet of the ground. They moved with remarkable rapidity over the surface of the wood, seeming to glide rather than run. Then an extra large and pungent cloud of smoke burst upwards and spread over them, and they decided to take to the air.

I have seen some extraordinary sights at one time and another, but the flight of the flying mice I shall remember until my dying day. The great tree was bound round with shifting columns of grey smoke that turned to the most ethereal blue where the great bars of sunlight stabbed through it. Into this the *Idiurus* launched themselves. They left the trunk of the tree without any apparent effort at jumping; one minute they were clinging spread-eagled to the bark, the next they were in the air. Their tiny legs were stretched out, and the membranes along their sides were taut. They swooped and drifted through the tumbling clouds of smoke with all the assurance and skill of hawking swallows, twisting and banking with incredible skill and apparently little or no movement of the body. This was pure gliding, and what they achieved was astonishing. I saw one leave the trunk of the tree at a height of about thirty feet. He glided across the dell in a straight and steady swoop, and landed on a tree about a hundred and fifty feet away, losing little, if any, height in the process. Others left the trunk of the smoke-enveloped tree and glided round it in a series of diminishing spirals, to land on a portion of the trunk lower down. Some patrolled the tree in a series of S-shaped patterns, doubling back on their tracks with great smoothness and efficiency. Their wonderful ability in the air amazed me, for there was no breeze in the forest to set up the air currents I should have thought essential for such intricate manoeuvring.

I noticed that although a number of them had flown off into the forest the majority stayed on the main trunk, contenting themselves with taking short flights around it when the smoke got too dense. This gave me an idea; I put out the fire, and as the smoke gradually drifted and dispersed, the *Idiurus* that were on the tree all scuttled back inside. We gave them a few minutes to settle down, while I examined the ones we had caught. At the base of the tree we had captured eight females and four males; Jacob lowered his catch down from the smoke-filled

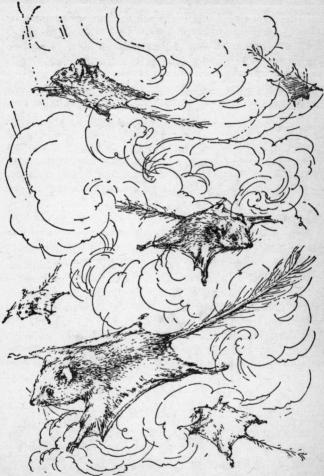

heavens, which consisted of two more males and one female. With them were two of the most extraordinary bats I had ever seen, with golden-brown backs and bright lemon-yellow shirt-fronts, faces like pigs and long, pig-like ears twisted down over their noses.

When the *Idiurus* had all returned to the tree we re-lit the fire, and once again they all rushed out. This time, however, they had grown wiser, and the majority refused to come anywhere near the nets at the main opening. Jacob, however, had better luck at the top of the tree, and soon lowered down a bag of twenty specimens, which I thought was quite enough to be getting on with. We put out the fire, removed the nets, got Jacob down from his tree-top perch (not without some difficulty, for he was very eager to try to catch the rest of the colony), and then we set off through the forest to walk the four odd miles that separated us from the village. I carried the precious bag of squeaking and scrambling *Idiurus* carefully in my hands, occasionally stopping to undo the top and fan them, for I was not at all sure they were getting sufficient air through the sides of the fine linen bag.

We reached the village, tired and dirty, just after dark. I put the *Idiurus* in the largest cage I had, but I found, to my annoyance, that it was far too small for such a great number. Stupidly, I had only banked on getting two or three *Idiurus*, if I got any at all, so had not brought a really large cage with me. I feared that if I left them in that confined space overnight the casualties in the morning would be heavy; there was only one thing to do, and that was to get the precious beasts back to the base camp as quickly as possible. I wrote a brief note to Smith, telling him that I had been successful and that I would be arriving some time about midnight with the animals, and would he please have a large cage ready for them. I sent this off at once, then I had a bath and some food. I reckoned that my letter would arrive at the camp about an hour before I did, which should give Smith plenty of time to improvise a cage.

About ten o'clock my little party started off along the Eshobi road. First walked Jacob carrying the lantern. Following him came a carrier with the box of *Idiurus* balanced on his woolly head. I was next in the row, and behind me was another carrier with my bed on his head. The Eshobi path is bad enough in broad daylight, but by night it is a death-trap. As a source of illumination the lantern was about as much use as an anaemic glow-worm; the light it gave was just sufficient to distort everything and to shroud rocks in deep shadow. Thus our progress was necessarily slow. Normally that walk would have taken us about two hours; that night it took us five. Most of the way I was on the edge of a nervous breakdown, for the carrier with the *Idiurus* hopped and jumped among the rocks like a mountain goat, and every minute I expected to see him slip and my precious box of specimens go hurtling into a ravine. He became more and more daring as the path got worse, until I felt that it was only a matter of time before he fell.

'My friend,' I called, 'if you go drop my beef, we no go reach Mamfe together. I go bury you here.'

He took the hint and slowed his progress considerably.

Half-way across a small stream my shadow got in the way of the carrier behind me, he missed his footing and stumbled and deposited my bed and bedding into the water with a loud splash. He was very upset about it, although I pointed out that it was mainly my fault. We continued on our way, the carrier with the dripping load on his head ejaculating at intervals 'Eh! Sorry, sah,' in a loud and doleful voice.

The forest around us was full of tiny sounds: the faint cracking of twigs, an occasional call from a frightened bird, the steady throbbing cry of the cicadas on the tree-trunks, and now and again a shrill piping from a tree-frog. The streams we crossed were ice-cold and transparent, and they whispered and licked at the big boulders in a conspiratorial fashion. At one point Jacob, up ahead, let out a loud yelp and started to dance around wildly, swinging the lamp so that the shadows writhed and twisted among the tree-trunks.

'Na whatee, na whatee?' called the carriers.

'Na ant,' said Jacob, still twirling round, 'blurry ant too much.'

Not looking where he was going, he had trodden straight in a column of Driver ants crossing the path, a black stream of them two inches wide that poured from the undergrowth on one side of the path and into that on the other side like a steady, silent river of tar. As his foot came down on them, the whole line seemed to boil up suddenly and silently, and within a second the ants were swarming over the ground in a horde, spreading further and further round the scene of the attack, like an inkstain on the brown leaves. The carriers and I had to make a detour into the forest to avoid their ferocious attentions.

As we left the shelter of the forest and walked out into the first moon-silvered grassfield, it started to rain. At first it was a fine drifting drizzle, more like mist; then, without warning, the sky let down a seemingly solid deluge of water, that bent the grass flat and turned the path into a treacherous slide of red mud. Fearing that my precious box of specimens would get drenched, and the *Idiurus* die in consequence, I took off my coat and draped it over the cage on the carrier's head. It was not much protection, but it helped. We struggled on, up to our ankles in mud, until we came to the river which we had to ford. Crossing this took us, I suppose, roughly three minutes, but it was quite long enough, for the carrier with the *Idiurus* on his head stumbled and staggered over the rocky bed, while the current plucked and pushed at him, waiting an opportunity to catch him off balance. But we arrived intact on the opposite bank, and soon we saw the lights of the camp gleaming through the trees. Just as we got to the marquee the rain stopped.

The cage that Smith had prepared for the *Idiurus* was not really large enough, but I felt that the main thing was to get the creatures out of the box they were in as soon as possible, for it was dripping like a newly emerged submarine. Carefully we undid the door and stood watching with bated breath as the tiny animals scuttled into their new home. None appeared to have got wet, which relieved me, though one or two of them looked a bit the worse for wear after the journey.

'What do they eat?' inquired Smith, when we had gloated over them for five minutes.

'I haven't the faintest idea. The one I caught yesterday didn't eat anything, though God knows I gave him enough choice.'

'Um, I expect they'll eat when they settle down a bit.'

'Oh, yes, I think they will,' I said cheerfully, and I really believed it.

We filled the cage with every form of food and drink there was to be had in camp, until it looked like a native market.

Then we hung a sack over the front of the cage and left the *Idiurus* to eat. My bed having absorbed rain and river water like a sponge, I was forced to spend a most uncomfortable night dozing in an upright camp chair. I slept fitfully until dawn, when I got up and hobbled over to the *Idiurus* cage, lifted the sacking and peered inside.

On the floor, among the completely untouched food and drink, lay a dead *Idiurus*. The others clung to the top of the cage like a flock of bats and twittered suspiciously at me. I retrieved the dead specimen and carried it over to the table, where I subjected it to a careful dissection. The stomach, to my complete surprise, was crammed with the partially digested red husk of the palm-nut. This was the very last thing I expected to find, for the palm-nut is, in the Cameroons at any rate, a cultivated product, and does not grow wild in the forest. If the rest of the colony had been eating palm-nuts on the night before they were captured by us, it meant that they must have travelled some four miles to the nearest native farm, and then come down to within a few feet of the ground to feed. This was all very puzzling, but at any rate it gave me something to work on, so the next night the *Idiurus* cage was festooned like a Christmas tree with bunches of red palm-nuts, in addition to the other foods. We put the food in at dusk, and for the next three hours Smith and I carried on long conversations that had nothing to do with *Idiurus*, and with an effort we pretended not to hear the squeaks and rustlings that came from their cage. After we had eaten, however, the strain became too great, and we crept up to the cage and gently lifted a corner of the sacking.

The entire colony of *Idiurus* was down on the floor of the cage, and all of them were busily engaged in eating palm-nuts. They squatted on their haunches and held the nuts in their minute pink forepaws like squirrels, turning the nuts quickly as their teeth shredded off the scarlet rind. They stopped eating as we lifted the sacking and peered at us; one or two of the more timid ones dropped their nuts and fled to the top of the cage, but the majority decided that we were harmless and continued to eat. We lowered the sacking into place and executed a war dance round the marquee, uttering loud cries to indicate our pleasure, cries that awoke the monkeys and set them chattering a protest and brought the staff tumbling out of the kitchen to see what was the matter. When they heard the good news that the new beef was chopping at last, they grinned and cracked their knuckles with pleasure, for they took our work very much to heart. All day gloom had pervaded the camp because the new beef would not chop, but now everything was all right, so the staff returned to the kitchen, chattering and laughing.

But our joy was short-lived, for on going to the cage next morning we found two *Idiurus* dead. From then on our little colony diminished steadily, week by week. They would eat only palm-nuts, and, apparently, this was not enough for them. It was quite astonishing the variety of food we put in the cage, and which they refused – astonishing because even with the most finicky animal you will generally strike something it likes, if you offer it a wide enough choice of food. It appeared that the *Idiurus* were not going to be easy to get back to England.

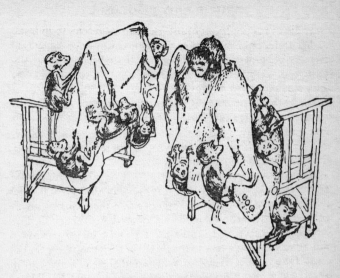

CHAPTER TWELVE

A Wilderness of Monkeys

PERHAPS the most noisy, the most irritating, and the most
lovable creatures that shared our marquee were the monkeys.
There were forty of them altogether, and life under the same
roof with forty monkeys is anything but quiet. The adult animals were not so bad; it was the baby monkeys that caused so
much trouble and extra work for us; they would scream
loudly if left alone, demand bottles full of warm milk at the
most ungodly hours of night and morning; they would get
stricken with all sorts of baby complaints and frighten us to
death; they would escape from the nursery and get near the
Golden Cat's cage, or fall into kerosene tins full of water, and
generally drive us to the edge of a nervous breakdown. We
were forced to think up the most Machiavellian schemes for
dealing with these babies, and some of them were quite extraordinary. Take the case of the baby Drills; these baboons are
extremely common in the forests of the Cameroons, and we

were always being brought babies of all ages. The Drill is that rather ugly-looking creature you can see in most zoos, who has a bright pink behind and does not hesitate to share its glory with you. Very young Drills are among the most pathetic and ridiculous-looking creatures in the world. they are covered with a very fine silvery grey fur, and their heads, hands, and feet look at least three times too big for their bodies. The hands, feet and face are a shade that we used to describe as boiled baby pink, and their minute bottoms were the same colour. The skin on their bodies was white, spotted in places with large areas, exactly like big birth-marks, of bright china blue. Like all baby monkeys, they have staring eyes, and their arms and legs are long and attenuated and tremble like the limbs of a very old person. This should give you some idea of a baby Drill.

The early days of a Drill's life are spent clinging with its muscular hands and feet to the thick fur of its mother. So our baby Drills, when they had transferred their affections to us and decided that we were their parents, demanded loudly and vociferously that they should be allowed to cling to us. Next to vast quantities of food, the most important thing in a young Drill's life is to feel that it has a good grip on the provider of the food. As it is almost impossible to work when you have four or five baby Drills clinging to you like miniature, cackling Old Men of the Sea, we had to devise some plan to keep them happy. We found two old coats and slung these over the backs of chairs in the centre of the marquee; then we introduced the babies to them. They were used to seeing us in these coats, and I expect the garments retained a certain characteristic odour, so they apparently decided that the coats were a sort of skin that we had discarded. They clung to the empty sleeves, the lapels, and the tails of these two coats as though they had been glued on, and while we went on with our work around the camp they would hang there, half asleep, occasionally waking up to carry on a cackling conversation with us.

The great numbers of people who used to visit our camp-site and look round the collection always seemed most affected by our group of baby monkeys. A baby monkey, in all its ways, is very like a human baby, only infinitely more pathetic.

The women in these parties would gaze at our young monkeys with melting eyes, making inarticulate crooning noises and generally brimming over with mother love. There was one young lady who visited us several times and was so affected by the pathetic expressions of the young monkeys that she unwisely took it upon herself to deliver a lecture to me about the extreme cruelty of taking these poor little creatures from their mothers and incarcerating them in cages. She waxed quite poetical on the joys of freedom, and contrasted the carefree, happy existence these babies would have in the tree-tops with the ghastly imprisonment for which I was responsible. That morning a baby monkey had been brought in by a native hunter, and since the young lady seemed to be such an expert on monkey life in the tree-tops, I suggested that she might like to help me perform a little task that had to be gone through with each new monkey that arrived. She agreed eagerly, seeing herself in the role of a sort of simian Florence Nightingale.

The little task consisted, quite simply, in searching the new baby for internal and external parasites. I explained this, and the young lady looked surprised: she said that she did not know that monkeys had parasites – beyond fleas, of course. I produced the little basket that the monkey was brought in, and removing some of its excreta I spread it out on a clean piece of paper and showed her the numbers of threadlike worms it contained. My helper remained strangely silent. Then I brought out the baby: he was a Putty-nose Guenon, an adorable little fellow clad in black fur, with a white shirt-front and a gleaming, heart-shaped patch of white fur on his nose. I examined his tiny hands and feet and his long slender fingers and toes and found no fewer than six jiggers comfortably ensconced. These minute creatures burrow their way into the skin of the feet and hands, particularly under the nails, where the skin is soft, and there they eat and swell and grow, until they reach the size of a match-head. Then they lay their eggs and die; in due course the eggs hatch and the baby jiggers continue the good work that their parent had begun. If a jigger infection is not dealt with in the early stages it can lead to the loss of the joint of a toe or finger, and in extreme cases it can destroy all the toes or fingers, for the jiggers go on burrowing and breeding until they have hollowed the part out to a bag of skin filled with pus. I have had jiggers in my foot on several occasions, and can vouch for the fact that they can be extremely painful. All this I explained to my helper in graphic detail. Then I got the tube of local anaesthetic, froze the fingers and toes of the little Guenon, and with a sterilized needle proceeded to remove the jiggers and disinfect the wounds they left. I found this local anaesthetic a boon, for the operation is painful and the baby monkeys would not sit still otherwise.

When this was over I ran my fingers down the monkey's tail and felt two sausage-shaped swellings, each as long as the first joint of my little finger and about the same circumference. I showed these to my companion, and then parted the hair so that she could see the circular, porthole-like opening at the end of each swelling. Looking through this porthole into the interior of the swelling, you could see something white and loathsome moving. I explained, with my best Harley Street air, that a certain forest fly lays its eggs on the fur of various animals, and when the maggot hatches it burrows down into the flesh of its host and lives there, fattening like a pig in a sty, getting air through the porthole, and, when it finally leaves to turn into a fly, the host has a hole the circumference of a cigarette in its flesh, which generally becomes a suppurating sore. I showed my helper, who was by now quite pale, that it was impossible to hook these maggots out. I got the needle and, parting the hair, showed her the creature lying in its burrow like a miniature barrage ballon; as soon as the tip of the needle touched it, however, it just compressed itself into a wrinkled blob, folding up like a concertina, and slid back into the depths of the monkey's tail. Then I showed her how to get them out – a method I had invented: pushing the nozzle of the anaesthetic tube into the porthole, I squirted the liquid inside until I had frozen the maggot into immobility; then, with a scalpel, I enlarged the porthole slightly, stabbed the maggot with the end of the needle and withdrew it from its lair. As I pulled the wrinkled white horror out of the blood-stained hole, my helper left me suddenly and precipitately. I

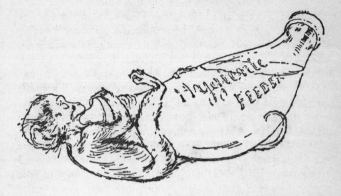

removed the second maggot, disinfected the gaping holes they had left and then joined her at the other side of the camp clearing. She explained that she was late for a lunch date, thanked me for a most interesting morning, and took her leave, never to visit us again. I always think it rather a pity that people don't learn more about the drawbacks of life in the jungle before prating about the cruelty of captivity.

One of the most delightful monkeys we had was a baby moustached Guenon, whom Smith procured on a trip up-country. He was the smallest monkey I had ever seen, and, except for his long slender tail, he could fit comfortably into a tea-cup. He was a greenish-grey in colour, with buttercup-yellow cheek-patches and a white shirt-front. But the most remarkable thing about him was his face, for across his upper lip was a broad, curving band of white hair that made him look as though he had an impressive moustache. For his size, his mouth was enormous, and could quite easily accommodate the teat of the feeding-bottle. It was a most amusing sight to see this tiny, moustached animal hurl himself on to the bottle when it arrived, uttering shrill squeaks of joy, wrap his arms and legs round it tightly, and lie there with his eyes closed, sucking away frantically. It looked rather as though he was being suckled by a large white airship, for the bottle was three times his size. He was very quick to learn, and it was not long before we had taught him to drink his milk out of a saucer. He would be put on the camp table to be fed, and the moment he saw the saucer approaching he would get quite hysterical with excitement, trembling and twitching, and screaming at the top of his voice. As soon as the saucer was placed before him he would, without any hesitation, dive head first into it. He would push his face completely under the milk, and only come up for air when he could hold out no longer. Sometimes, in his greed, he would wait too long, and a shower of bubbles would break the surface, and he would follow them, coughing and sneezing and spattering himself and the table with a fountain of milk. There were times during his meal when he would become convinced that you were hanging around waiting an opportunity to take his saucer away from him, and, giving a quavering scream of rage, he would frustrate your plan by the simple expedient of leaping into the air and landing in the centre of the saucer with a splash, where he would sit glaring at you triumphantly. At meal-times he would get his head and face so covered with milk that it was only with difficulty you could tell where his moustache began and ended, and the table would look as though someone had milked a large and healthy cow over it.

The two most forceful characters in our monkey collection were, of course, the chimpanzees Mary and Charlie. Charlie had been the pet of a planter before he came to us, so he was fairly domesticated. He had a small, wrinkled, sorrowful face and melting brown eyes; he looked as though the world had treated him harshly but that he was too much of a saint to complain. This wounded, dejected air was a lot of moonshine, for in reality Charlie, far from being an ill-treated, misunderstood ape, was a disgraceful little street urchin, full of low cunning and deceit. Every day we used to let him out of his cage for exercise, and he would roam about the camp looking radiantly innocent until he thought he had lulled you into believing in his integrity. Then he would wander nonchalantly towards the food-table, give a quick glance round to see if he was observed, grab the largest bunch of bananas within reach, and dash madly away towards the nearest tree. If you gave chase he would drop the fruit and skid to a standstill. Then he would sit in

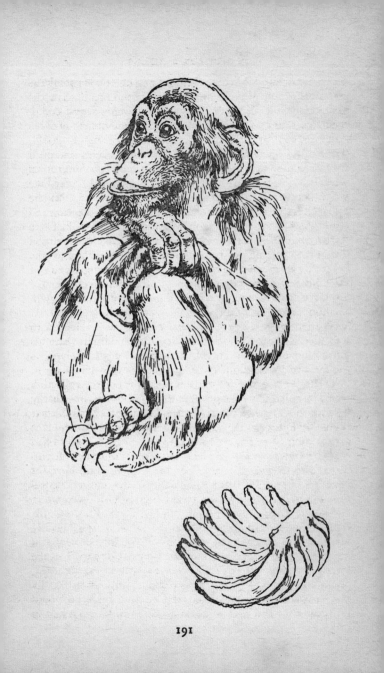

the dust while you scolded him, gazing up at you sorrowfully, the picture of injured innocence, the expression on his face showing quite plainly that he was being wrongfully accused of a monstrous crime, but that he was far too noble to point that out to you if you were too obtuse to realize it. Wave the bunch of stolen fruit under his nose and he would regard it with faint surprise, mingled with disgust. Why should you imagine that he had stolen the fruit? his expression seemed to say. Were you not aware of the fact that he disliked bananas? Never in his whole life (devoted to philanthropy and self-denial) had he felt the slightest inclination to even sample the loathsome fruit, much less steal any. The scolding over, Charlie would rise, give a deep sigh, throw you a look of compassion tinged with disgust, and lope off to the kitchen to see what he could steal there. He was quite incorrigible, and his face was so expressive that he could carry on a long conversation with you without any need of speech.

Charlie's greatest triumph came when we received a visit from the High Commissioner for the Cameroons, who was passing through on one of his periodical visits of inspection. He came down to our camp accompanied by a vast army of secretaries and other supporters, and was greatly interested in our large array of beasts. But the animal that attracted him most was Charlie. While we explained to H.E. what a disgusting hypocrite the ape was, Charlie was sitting in his cage, holding the great man's hand through the bars, and gazing up at him with woe-begone expression and pleading eyes, begging that His Excellency would not listen to the foul slander we were uttering. When His Excellency left, he invited Smith and myself to his At Home, which was to take place the following evening. The next morning a most impressive messenger, glittering with golden buttons, delivered an envelope from the District Office. Inside was a large card which informed us, in magnificent twirly writing, that His Excellency, the High Commissioner for the Cameroons, requested the pleasure of Charlie's presence during his At Home, between the hours of six and eight. When we showed it to Charlie he was sitting in his cage meditating, and he gave it a brief glance and then ignored it. His attitude told us he was quite used to being showered with such invitations, but that these things were too worldly to be of any interest to him. He was, he implied, far too busy with his saint-like meditations to get excited about invitations to drinking-orgies with mere High Commissioners. As he had been into the kitchen that morning and stolen six eggs, a loaf of bread, and a leg of cold chicken, we did not believe him.

Mary was a chimp of completely different character. She was older than Charlie, and much bigger, being about the size of a two-year-old human. Before we bought her she had been in the hands of a Hausa trader, and I am afraid she must have been teased and ill-treated, for at first she was sullen and vicious, and we feared we would never be able to gain her confidence as she had developed a deep-rooted mistrust of anything human, black or white. But after a few months of good food and kind handling she delighted us by blossoming forth into a chimp with much charm, a sunny disposition and a terrific sense of humour. She had a pale pink, rather oafish face, and a large pot belly. She reminded me rather of a fat barmaid, who was always ready to laugh uproariously at some bawdy jest. After she got to know and trust us, she developed a trick which she thought was frightfully funny. She would lie back in her cage, balanced precariously on her perch, and present an unmentionable part of her anatomy to the bars. You were then expected to lean forward and blow hard whereupon Mary would utter a screech of laughter and modestly cover herself up with her hands. Then she would give you a coy look from over the mound of her stomach, and uncover herself again and you were expected to repeat the mirth-provoking action. This became known to both us and the staff as Blowing Mary's Wicked Parts, and no matter how many times a day you repeated it, Mary still found it exceedingly funny; she would throw back her head and open her mouth wide, showing vast areas of pink gum and white teeth, hooting and tittering with hysterical laughter.

Although Mary treated us and the staff with great gentleness, she never forgot that she had a grudge against Africans in general, and she used to pick on any strange ones that came to camp. She would grin at them ingratiatingly and slap her chest, or turn somersaults – anything to gain their attention. By her antics she would lure them closer and closer to the cage looking the picture of cheerful good humour, while her shrewd eyes judged the distance carefully. Suddenly the long and powerful arm would shoot out through the bars, there would be a loud ripping noise, a yelp of fright from the African, and Mary would be dancing round her cage triumphantly waving a torn shirt or singlet that she had pulled off her admirer's back. Her strength was extraordinary, and it cost me a small fortune in replacements until I put her cage in such a position that she could not commit these outrages.

The monkey collection kept up a continuous noise all through the day, but in the afternoon, at about four-thirty, this rose to a crescendo of sound that would tax the strongest nerves, for it was at this time that the monkeys had their milk. About four they would start to get impatient, leaping and jumping about their cages, turning somersaults, or sitting with their faces pressed to the bars making mournful squeaks. As soon as the line of clean pots was laid out, however, and the great kerosene tin full of warm milk, malt and cod-liver oil, sugar and calcium came in sight, a wave of excitement would sweep the cages and the uproar would be deafening. The chimps would be giving prolonged hoots through pursed lips and thumping on the sides of their cages with their fists, the Drills would be uttering their loud and penetrating 'Ar-ar-ar-ar-ar-erererer!' cries, like miniature machine-guns, the Guenons would be giving faint, bird-like whistles and trills, the Patas monkeys would be dancing up and down like mad ballerinas, shouting 'Proup ... proup' plaintively, and the beautiful Colobus, with her swaying shawl of white and black hair, would be calling 'Arroup! arroup! arroup! ye-ye-ye-ye!' in a commanding tone of voice. As we moved along the cages, pushing the pots of milk through the doors, the noises would gradually cease, until all that could be heard was a low snorting, sucking sound, interspersed by an occasional cough as some milk went down the wrong way. Then, the pots empty, the monkeys would climb up on to their perches and sit there, their bellies bulging, uttering loud and satisfied belches at regular intervals. After a while they would all climb down again on to the floor to examine their pots and make quite sure there was no milk left in them, even picking them up and looking underneath. Then they would curl up on their perches in the evening sun and fall into a bloated stupor, while peace came to the camp.

One of the things that I find particularly endearing about monkeys is the fact that they are completely uninhibited, and will perform any action they feel like with an entire lack of embarrassment. They will urinate copiously, or bend down and watch their own faeces appear with expressions of absorbed interest; they will mate or masturbate with great freedom, regardless of any audience. I have heard embarrassed human beings call monkeys dirty, filthy creatures when they have watched them innocently perform these actions in public, and it is an attitude of mind that I always find difficult to understand. After all, it is we, with our superior intelligence, who have decided that the perfectly natural functions of our bodies are something unclean; monkeys do not share our view.

Similarly, one of the things I liked about the Africans was this same innocent attitude towards the functions of the body. In this respect they were extremely like the monkeys. I had a wonderful example of this one day when a couple of rather stuffy missionaries came to look round the camp.

I showed them our various animals and birds, and they made a lot of unctuous comments about them. Then we came to the monkeys, and the missionaries were delighted with them. Presently, however, we reached a cage where a monkey was sitting on the perch in a curious hunched-up attitude.

'Oh! What's *he* doing?' cried the lady gaily, and before I could prevent her she had bent down to get a better look. She shot up again, her face a deep, rich scarlet, for the monkey had been whiling away the hours to meal time by sitting there and sucking himself.

We hurried through the rest of the monkey collection in record time, and I was much amused by the expression of frozen disgust that had replaced the look of benevolent delight on the lady missionary's face. They might be God's creatures, her expression implied, but she wished He would do something about their habits. However, as we rounded the corner of the marquee we were greeted by another of God's creatures in the shape of a lanky African hunter. He was a man who had brought in specimens regularly each week, but for the past fortnight he had not come near us.

'Iseeya, Samuel!' I greeted him.

'Iseeya, Masa,' he said, coming towards us.

'Which side you done go all dis time?' I asked; 'why you never bring me beef for two weeks, eh?'

'Eh! Masa, I done get sickness,' he explained.

'Sickness? Eh, sorry, my friend. Na what sickness you get?'

'Na my ghonereah, Masa,' he explained innocently, 'my ghonereah de worry me *too much*.'

The missionaries were among the people who never called twice at the camp site.

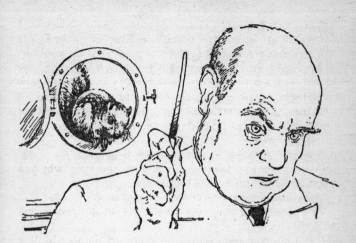

In Which we Walka Good

THE last few days before you and the collection join the ship
that is to take you back to England are always the most hectic
of the whole trip. There are a thousand things that have to be
done: lorries to hire, cages to strengthen, vast quantities of
food to be purchased and crated up, and all this on top of the
normal routine work of maintaining the collection.

One of the things that worried us most were the *Idiurus*.
Our colony had by now diminished to four specimens, and
we were determined to try to get them safely back to England.
We had, after superhuman efforts, got them to eat avocado
pears as well as palm-nuts, and on this diet they seemed to do
quite well. I decided that if we took three dozen avocados with
us, in varying stages from ripe to green, there would be enough
to last the voyage and with some left over to use in England
while the *Idiurus* were settling down. Accordingly, I called
Jacob and informed him that he must procure three dozen
avocados without delay. To my surprise, he looked at me as
though I had taken leave of my senses.

'Avocado pear, sah?' he asked.

197

'Yes, avocado pear,' I said.

'I no fit get 'um sah,' he said mournfully.

'You no fit get 'um? Why not?'

'Avocado pear done finish,' said Jacob helplessly.

'Finish? What you mean, finish? I want you go for market and get 'um, not from kitchen.'

'Done finish for market, sah,' said Jacob patiently.

Suddenly it dawned on me what he was trying to explain: the season for avocado pears had finished, and he could not get me any. I would have to face the voyage with no supply of the fruit for the precious *Idiurus*.

It was just like the *Idiurus*, I reflected bitterly, to start eating something when it was going out of season. However, avocados I had to have, so in the few days at our disposal I marshalled the staff and made them scour the countryside for the fruit. By the time we were ready to move down country we had obtained a few small, shrivelled avocados, and that was all. These almost mummified remains had to last my precious *Idiurus* until we reached England.

We had to travel some two hundred miles down to the coast from our base camp, and it required three lorries and a small van to carry our collection. We travelled by night, for it was cooler for the animals, and the journey took us two days. It was one of the worst journeys I can ever remember. We had to stop the lorries every three hours, take out all the frog-boxes, and sprinkle them with cold water to prevent them drying up. Twice during each night we had to make prolonged stops to bottle-feed the young animals on warm milk which we carried ready mixed in thermos flasks. Then, when dawn came, we had to pull the lorries into the side of the road under the shade of the great trees, unload every single cage on to the grass and clean and feed every specimen. On the morning of the third day we arrived at the small rest-house on the coast which had been put at our disposal; here everything had to be unpacked once again and cleaned and fed before we could crawl into the house, eat a meal, and collapse on our beds to sleep. That evening parties of people from the local banana plantations came round to see the animals and, half dead with sleep, we were forced to conduct tours, answer questions and be polite.

'Are you travelling on this ship that's in?' inquired someone.

'Yes,' I said, stifling a yawn; 'sailing tomorrow.'

'Good Lord! I pity you, then,' they said cheerfully.

'Oh. Why is that?'

'Captain's a bloody Tartar, old boy, and he hates animals. It's a fact. Old Robinson wanted to take his pet baboon back with him on this ship when he went on leave last time. Captain chucked it off. Wouldn't have it on board. Said he didn't want his ship filled with stinking monkeys. Frightful uproar about it, so I heard.'

Smith and I exchanged anxious looks, for of all the evils that can befall a collector, an unsympathetic captain is perhaps the worst. Later, when the last party of sightseers had gone, we discussed this disturbing bit of news. We decided that we should have to go out of our way to be polite to the Captain; and we would take extra care to make sure there were no untoward incidents among the monkeys to earn his wrath.

Our collection was placed on the forward deck under the supervision of the Chief Officer, a most charming and helpful man. The Captain we did not see that night, and the next morning, when we arose early to clean out the cages, we could see him pacing on the bridge, a hunched and terrifying figure. We had been told that he would be down to breakfast, and we were looking forward to meeting him with some trepidation.

'Remember,' said Smith as we cleaned out the monkeys, 'we must keep on the right side of him.' He filled a basket full of sawdust, trotted to the rail and cast it into the sea.

'We must be careful not to do anything that will annoy him,' he went on when he had returned.

Just at that moment a figure in spotless white uniform came running breathlessly down from the bridge.

'Excuse me, sir,' he said, 'but the Captain's compliments, sir, and will you please make sure which way the wind's blowing before you chuck that sawdust overboard?'

Horror-stricken, we looked up towards the bridge: the air was full of swirling fragments of sawdust, and the Captain, scowling angrily, was brushing his bespattered uniform.

'Please apologize to the Captain for us,' I said, conquering a frightful desire to laugh. When the officer had gone, I turned to Smith.

'Keep on the right side of him!' I said bitterly; 'don't do anything to annoy him! Only fling about three hundredweight of sawdust all over him and his precious bridge. Trust you to know the right way to a captain's heart.'

When the gong sounded we hurried down to our cabin, washed, and took our seats in the dining-saloon. We found, to our dismay, that we were seated at the Captain's table. The Captain sat with his back to the bulkhead, in which there were three portholes, and Smith and I sat on the opposite side of the circular table. The portholes behind the Captain's chair looked out into the well-deck in which our collection was stacked. Half-way through the meal the Captain had thawed out a little and was even starting to make tolerant little jokes about sawdust.

'As long as you don't let anything escape, I don't mind,' he said jovially, disembowelling a fried egg.

'Oh, we won't let that happen,' I said, and the words were hardly out of my mouth when something moved in the porthole, and, glancing up, there was Sweeti-pie, the Black-eared Squirrel, perched in the opening, examining the inside of the saloon with a kindly eye.

The Captain, of course, could not see the squirrel sitting on a level with his shoulder and about three feet away, and he went on eating and talking unconcernedly, while behind him Sweeti-pie sat on his hind legs and cleaned his whiskers. For a few seconds I was so startled that my brain refused to function, and I could only sit there gaping at the porthole. Luckily the Captain was too intent on his breakfast to notice. Sweeti-pie finished his wash and brush-up, and began to look round the saloon again. He decided that the place would be worth investigating, and glanced around to see which was the best way to get down from his perch. He decided that the quickest method would be to jump from the porthole on to the Captain's shoulder. I could see this plan taking shape in the little brute's head, and the thought of his landing on the Captain's shoulder galvanized me into action. Muttering a hasty 'Excuse me', I pushed back my chair and walked out of the saloon; as soon as I was out of sight of the Captain I ran as fast as I could out on to the deck. To my relief, Sweeti-pie had not jumped, and his long bushy tail was still hanging outside the porthole. I flung myself across the hatch-cover and grabbed him by his tail just as he bunched himself up to spring. I bundled him, chattering indignantly, into his cage, and then returned, flushed but triumphant, to the saloon. The Captain was still talking and, if he had noticed my abrupt departure at all, must have attributed it to the pangs of nature, for he made no mention of it.

On the third day of the voyage two of the *Idiurus* were dead. I was examining their corpses sorrowfully when a member of the crew appeared. He asked why the little animals had died, and I explained at great length the tragic tale of the non-existent avocado pears.

'What's an avocado pear?' he inquired.

I showed him one of the shrivelled wrecks.

'Oh, *those* things,' he said. 'Do you want some?'

I gazed at him speechlessly for a minute.

'Have you got some?' I said at last.

'Well,' he said, 'I haven't exactly got any, but I think I can get you some.'

That evening he reappeared with his pockets bulging.

'Here,' he said, stuffing some beautifully ripe avocados into my hand; 'give me three of those ones of yours, and don't say a word to anyone.'

I gave him three of my dried-up fruits and hastily fed the *Idiurus* with the ripe ones he had procured, and they enjoyed them thoroughly. My spirits rose, and I began to have hopes once more of landing them in England.

My sailor friend brought me plump, ripe avocados whenever I informed him that my stock was running low, and always he took some of my desiccated stock in exchange. It was very

curious, but I felt the best thing I could do was not to inquire
too deeply into the matter. However, in spite of the fresh fruit,
another *Idiurus* died, so by the time we were rolling through
the Bay of Biscay I had only one specimen left. It was now, I
realized, a fight against time: if I could keep this solitary specimen alive until we reached England, I would have a tremendous variety of food to offer it, and I felt sure that I could find
something it would eat. As we drew closer and closer to England I watched the little chap carefully. He seemed fit, and in
the best spirits. As an additional precaution, I smuggled his
cage into my cabin each night, so that he would not catch a
chill. The day before we docked he was in fine fettle, and I
became almost convinced that I would land him. That night,
quite suddenly and for no apparent reason, he died. So, after
travelling four thousand miles, the last *Idiurus* died twenty-four
hours out of Liverpool. I was bitterly disappointed, and black
depression settled on me.

Even the sight of the collection being taken ashore did not
fill me with the usual mixture of relief and pride. The Hairy
Frogs had come through, as had the Brow-leaf Toads;
Charlie and Mary were hooting in their cages as they were
swung overboard. Sweeti-pie was eating a sugar-lump and
eyeing the crowd on the docks with hopeful eyes, while the
Moustached Monkey peered from his cage, his whiskers
gleaming, looking like a juvenile Santa Claus. But even the
sight of all these creatures being landed safely after so long and
so dangerous a trip did not altogether compensate me for the
loss of my little *Idiurus*, and Smith and I were just going to
leave the ship when my sailor friend appeared. He had heard
the news about *Idiurus*, and was extremely upset to think that
our combined efforts had been in vain.

'By the way,' I said, just as I was leaving him, 'I am very
curious to know where you got those avocado pears from in
mid-ocean.'

He glanced round to make sure we were not overheard.

'I'll tell you, mate; only keep it under your hat,' he said in
a hoarse whisper. 'The Captain's very partial to an avocado,
see, and he has a big box of them in the fridge. He always

brings home a box, see? I just got some of them for you.'

'Do you mean to say those were the Captain's avocados?' I asked faintly.

'Sure. But he won't miss 'em,' my friend assured me cheerfully; 'you see, every time I took some of *his* out I put the same number of *yours* back in the box.'

The customs men could not understand why I kept shaking with laughter as I was showing them our crates, and they kept darting suspicious looks at me. But it was not, unfortunately, the sort of joke you could share.

FOR THE BEST IN PAPERBACKS, LOOK FOR THE 🐧

In every corner of the world, on every subject under the sun, Penguin represents quality and variety – the very best in publishing today.

For complete information about books available from Penguin – including Pelicans, Puffins, Peregrines and Penguin Classics – and how to order them, write to us at the appropriate address below. Please note that for copyright reasons the selection of books varies from country to country.

In the United Kingdom: For a complete list of books available from Penguin in the U.K., please write to *Dept E.P., Penguin Books Ltd, Harmondsworth, Middlesex, UB7 0DA*

In the United States: For a complete list of books available from Penguin in the U.S., please write to *Dept BA, Penguin, 299 Murray Hill Parkway, East Rutherford, New Jersey 07073*

In Canada: For a complete list of books available from Penguin in Canada, please write to *Penguin Books Canada Ltd, 2801 John Street, Markham, Ontario L3R 1B4*

In Australia: For a complete list of books available from Penguin in Australia, please write to the *Marketing Department, Penguin Books Australia Ltd, P.O. Box 257, Ringwood, Victoria 3134*

In New Zealand: For a complete list of books available from Penguin in New Zealand, please write to the *Marketing Department, Penguin Books (NZ) Ltd, Private Bag, Takapuna, Auckland 9*

In India: For a complete list of books available from Penguin, please write to *Penguin Overseas Ltd, 706 Eros Apartments, 56 Nehru Place, New Delhi, 110019*

In Holland: For a complete list of books available from Penguin in Holland, please write to *Penguin Books Nederland B.V., Postbus 195, NL–1380AD Weesp, Netherlands*

In Germany: For a complete list of books available from Penguin, please write to *Penguin Books Ltd, Friedrichstrasse 10 – 12, D–6000 Frankfurt Main 1, Federal Republic of Germany*

In Spain: For a complete list of books available from Penguin in Spain, please write to *Longman Penguin España, Calle San Nicolas 15, E–28013 Madrid, Spain*

An Appeal by Gerald Durrell

JERSEY WILDLIFE PRESERVATION TRUST

Have you enjoyed this Book?

If you have, it is the animals that have made this possible; and these animals are not just characters in a book: They *really* exist. But many of them will not exist for much longer unless they have your help.

All over the world the wildlife that I wrote about is in grave danger. It is being exterminated by what we call the progress of civilization. A great number of creatures will become extinct in a very short time if something is not done, and done swiftly.

Some years ago I created on the Island of Jersey a zoological park which is now the headquarters of the Jersey Wildlife Preservation Trust. Our aim is to create a sanctuary in which we can establish breeding colonies of these threatened species, so that, even if they become extinct in the wild state, they will not vanish forever.

To do this work money is required.

Therefore we need as many members as possible to join the Trust. It will cost you little, but you will be helping a cause that is of the utmost importance and urgency. I say 'urgency' advisedly, because, as you read this, yet another species is added to the danger list.

If the animals I write about have given you pleasure, please join the Trust. The animals will be greatly indebted for every subscription received.

Full particulars can be obtained from:
      The Secretary,
      Jersey Wildlife Preservation Trust,
      Les Augres Manor,
      JERSEY,
      Channel Islands.

GERALD DURRELL

MY FAMILY AND OTHER ANIMALS
The family with its many eccentric hangers-on and the procession of animals Gerry brings back to the villas in Corfu are both described in the author's inimitably endearing manner.

THE DRUNKEN FOREST
The Argentine pampas and the little-known Chaco territory of Paraguay provide the setting for such exotic creatures as an orange armadillo or a crab-eating racoon.

ENCOUNTERS WITH ANIMALS
Uniquely entertaining accounts of the courtships, wars and characters of animals in West Africa and elsewhere.

A ZOO IN MY LUGGAGE
Here Gerald Durrell chronicles the birth of a private zoo – the collection of the animals and the problems of accommodating them.

THE WHISPERING LAND
The author searches windswept Patagonian shores and tropical forests in the Argentine for additions to his zoo.

THREE SINGLES TO ADVENTURE
On this trip to South America the reader meets the sakiwinki and the sloth clad in bright green fur, hears the horrifying sound of piranha fish on the rampage and learns how to lasso a galloping anteater.

MENAGERIE MANOR
With the help of an enduring wife, a selfless staff and a reluctant bank manager Gerald Durrell's private zoo on Jersey is able to expand.